Today's Herbal Health

3rd Edition

by

Louise Tenney, M.H.

Today's Herbal Health
3rd Edition

© 1992 by Louise Tenney, M.H.

Published by
Woodland Books
P.O. Box 1422
Provo, Utah

Printed in the United States of America

Contents

Dedicated

This book is dedicated to Josie, a dear friend who believes in Herbs, and has encouraged me every step of the way. She was my inspiration when it looked like this book would never come together.

Notice to the Reader

THIS HERBAL HEALTH BOOK IS NOT INTENDED TO PRESCRIBE OR DIAGNOSE IN ANY WAY. IT IS NOT MEANT TO BE A SUBSTITUTE FOR PROFESSIONAL HELP. THE INTENT IS TO OFFER HISTORICAL USES OF HERBS. THOSE WHO ARE SICK SHOULD CONSULT THEIR DOCTOR.
NEITHER THE AUTHOR NOR THE PUBLISHER DIRECTLY OR INDIRECTLY DISPENSE MEDICAL ADVICE OR PRESCRIBE THE USE OF HERBS AS A FORM OF TREATMENT. THE AUTHOR AND THE PUBLISHER ASSUME NO RESPONSIBILITY IF YOU PRESCRIBE FOR YOURSELF WITHOUT YOUR DOCTOR'S APPROVAL.

Introduction

Herbs are considered food for the body. If we desire a healthy body and mind we must search for the herb that will provide the essential nutrients that will supply our special needs.

Herbs are valuable sources of natural medicine, vitamins and minerals which have a remarkable history of curative effects, when used in the proper way. Every plant put on this earth has a purpose. Every part of this earth has herbs that provide a remedy for diseases that might afflict mankind. The herbs that are useful for certain ailments usually contain vitamins and minerals that are also helpful in that particular ailment. The more research I do on herbs the better appreciation I have for God's creations.

All the drugs which are extracted from plants are not used in their natural state. This is why we have so many side effects from prescribed medicines. Chemical drugs are not the answer. Every drug has some possible side-effect. The side-effects of drugs are increased even greater if a person has more than one ailment.

Most herbs in their natural state could be the answer. They are safe and do not leave built up residue in the system that produces side effects.

Herbs work best in a healthy, clean body. They work best

with a natural food diet. Everyone can benefit from using herbs, but the best results will be realized when the body is clean and free from built up toxins.

Herbalists realize that the body can heal itself. The essence of natural therapy is to activate the body's own self-healing powers. In other words Natural Therapy is the administration of a natural remedy, which allows the body to cure itself.

Orthodox medicine cannot change the working of the body, it can only help it. Many doctors believe that their patients get well because of drugs and surgery alone, and ignore the fact that the body has its own healing powers.

This book is for those who are interested in knowing why herbs, vitamins, minerals and natural foods work the way they do. No one wants to follow blindly old wives tales when it comes to the use of plants in medicine.

Science is discovering the wonderful properties of herbs, and their value to mankind. The day will come when herbal remedies will be able to fill all the needs of mankind.

Herbal Preparations

BOLUS

A bolus is a suppository to be used as an internal poultice in the rectal or vaginal area to help draw the toxic poisons to it or is the carrier for healing agents.

The bolus is made by adding powdered herbs to cocoa butter until it forms a thick, firm consistency. It is usually placed in the refrigerator to harden and then is brought to room temperature before using.

The bolus can be inserted into the rectum to treat hemorrhoids or cysts, or into the vagina to treat infections, irritations or tumors. The bolus is usually applied at night when the cocoa butter will melt with the body heat, thus releasing the herbs.

The herbs used in the bolus are usually astringents such as white oak bark or bayberry bark: demulcent healing herbs such as comfrey or slippery elm, and antibiotic herbs such as garlic, chaparral or golden seal.

CAPSULES

Gelatin capsules provide a pleasant way of taking herbs, especially when they are bitter-tasting or mucilaginous. Herbs such as goldenseal, mandrake, poke and lobelia should be taken

in smaller quantities and are usually mixed with other herbs.
    If the capsules are purchased from a first-class herb com-
pany they may be depended on to be clean and combined in the
right proportion. They are prepared and measured by chemists
trained in the herb field.
    To help in washing down and dissolving the capsules, they
should be taken with eight ounces of pure water or herbal tea.

COMPRESSES

    An herbal compress will achieve a similar effect as an
ointment with the advantage of the therapeutic action of heat.
One or two heaping tablespoons of the herb or herbs are brought
to a boil in 1 cup of water. A cotton pad or gauze is dipped in the
strained liquid, and the excess liquid is, drained off, then placed
on the affected area while still warm. Then it is best covered with
a piece of woolen material. For small children, it could be
bandaged into place. When cool, the compress is changed. Use
sterile gauze. Compresses are used in cases of injury, contusions,
and effusions.
    A compress is also known as a fomentation. This is used
when herbs that are too strong to be taken internally may be used
externally and will be absorbed in small amounts slowly into the
system.
    A compress is used to stimulate circulation of the blood or
lymph in the body. It is used for superficial ailments including
swellings, pains, colds and flu.
    A ginger compress may be used by grating two ounces of
fresh ginger root and squeezed into a pint of hot water until the
water turns yellow. Apply the compress, having an alternate
towel ready as soon as one cools. It can be used to stimulate
circulation of blood and lymph, to relieve colic, to reduce
internal inflammation and to restore warmth to cold joints.

DECOCTION

A decoction is used when a plant is not soluble in cold or boiling hot water, but will often yield its soluble ingredients by simmering in water five to twenty minutes. Five minutes is enough if the material is finely shredded. If the herb is hard or woody, twenty minutes is necessary to produce a good extract. It is more useful if the plants are first soaked in cold water and then brought to a boil.

A teaspoon of the dried herb is placed in an enamel or glass container with one cup of pure water. Decoctions should always be strained while hot so the ingredients which separate on cooling may be mixed again with the fluid by shaking when the remedy is used.

This method is valuable for extracting the essential mineral salts and alkaloids from the herbs.

EXTRACTS

Herbal extracts are rubbed into the skin for treating strained muscles and ligaments. Some are used for the relief of arthritis or other inflammation. They usually contain stimulating herbs, such as cayenne and antispasmodic herbs, like lobelia.

They can be made by putting four ounces of dried herbs or eight ounces of fresh bruised herbs into a jar. Add one pint of vinegar, alcohol or massage oil and allow to extract. Shake the bottle once or twice daily. It will take about four days, if the herbs are powdered and about 15 days if the herbs are whole or cut.

If oil such as olive or almond is used, a little vitamin E can be added for a preservative. The oil is useful where one wishes to use it for massage purposes.

The use of alcohol extract (Vodka or Gin) or rubbing alcohol (for external use only) will be somewhat cooling, allowing the liquid to evaporate quickly and leaving the herbs on the skin.

When the extracts are purchased from a first class herb company, they may be depended upon.

INFUSION

An infusion is made by pouring the hot liquid over the crude or powdered herb and steeping to extract their active ingredients. This method of preparation minimizes the loss of volatile elements. The usual amounts are about ½ to 1 oz. to a pint of water. Use an enamel, porcelain, or glass pot to steep the herbs fro about 10 to 20 minutes, then cover with a tight fitting lid to avoid evaporation. For drinking, strain the infusion into a cup. For general purposes, drink lukewarm or cool; but to induce sweating and to break up a cold or a cough, take it hot.

OINTMENTS

Ointments are used on the skin when the active principles of herbs are needed for extended periods and thus accelerate healing, as in cases of injury, contusion and effusion. There are vaseline products that are made from natural sources that can be used instead of petroleum products. One or two heaping table-spoons of the herb or herbs are brought to boil in the vaseline. The mixture is then stirred and strained. When cold, an ointment is put into jars and is ready for use when needed.

OILS

The herb oils are very useful when ointments or com-presses are not practical. Herb oils need to be stored in **brown glass containers.**

When the major properties of an herb are associated with its essential oils, an oil extract will prove to be a useful way of preparing a concentrate from fresh herbs. Oils are prepared by macerating and pounding the fresh or dried herbs. Olive oil or sesame oil is added (2 oz. of herb to one pint of oil) and the mixture is put in a warm place for about four days. A quicker method is to gently heat the oil and herbs in a pan for one hour. Then the oil is strained and bottled. A small amount of vitamin E is added to help preserve the preparation.

Oils are usually made from the aromatic herbs such as eucalyptus, peppermint, spearmint and spices.

POULTICE

A poultice is a warm mashed fresh or ground powdered herb that is applied directly to the skin to relieve inflammation, blood poisoning, venomous bites and eruptions, boils, and abscesses and to promote proper cleansing and healing of the affected area. Oil the skin before applying a hot poultice.

Comfrey, golden seal and aloe vera juice can be applied to bruises and a bandage put on for a few hours. Many herbs have the ingredients to draw out infections, toxins and foreign bodies embedded in the skin. Plantain and marshmallow are very good to relieve pain and muscle spasm. Cayenne (to stimulate) is added to herbs such as lobelia, valerian, catnip or echinacea. The powdered herbs are moistened with hot water, apple cider vinegar, herbal tea, a liniment, or a tincture. Apply antiseptic before applying poultice.

A plaster is like a poultice. An effective plaster for drawing out fever can be made by squeezing out the water from tofu and mashing with pastry flour and about 5 per cent fresh ginger root.

POWDERS

Powders are made from fresh plant parts and mashed until there are fine particles of the herbal agent. This way the herb can be taken in a capsule, in water, in herb teas, or sprinkled on food.

This is an ideal way to introduce herbs slowly and to become adjusted to the dosage.

For external use, the powdered herbs are mixed with oil, vaseline or petroleum jelly, or a little water or aloe vera juice and applied to the skin to treat wounds, inflammation, and contusions.

SALVES

Fresh or dried herbs are covered with water brought to a boil, then simmered for thirty minutes. This is then strained and added to an equal amount of olive oil or safflower oil. Simmer until the water has evaporated in steam and only the oil is left. Add enough beeswax to give the mixture salve consistency and pour into a dark glass jar with a tight lid. Salves will last a long time, up to a year.

SYRUPS

A syrup is ideal in treating coughs, mucus congestion, bronchial catarrh and sore throats because it will coat the area and keep the herbs in direct contact. Syrups are especially good for children and people with sensitive palates.

Syrups are made by adding about two ounces of herbs to a quart of water and gently boil down to one pint and while still warm, add two ounces of honey and/or glycerine. Licorice and wild cherry bark are commonly used as flavors and as therapeutic agents in making syrups. Other herbs used are comfrey, anise seed, fennel seed and Irish moss.

TINCTURE

Tinctures are solutions of concentrated herbal extracts that can be kept for long periods because the alcohol is a good preservative. Tinctures are useful for herbs that do not taste good or are to be taken over an extended period of time, and may be used externally as a liniment. Tinctures are usually made with more potent herbs that are generally not taken as herbal teas. Tinctures can be made by combining four ounces of powdered or cut herb with one pint of alcohol such as vodka, brandy, gin or rum. Shake daily, allowing the herbs to extract for about two weeks. Let the herbs settle and pour off the tincture, straining out the powder through cheese cloth. The extract can be made with vinegar. Tinctures are very convenient for external application.

SECTION II

Concentrated Herbs

Concentrated herbs are a great break through in the field of natural medicine. We have concentrated vitamins, so why not herbs? Like vitamins, some herbs need to be taken in larger doses to be effective. For people who take large numbers of capsules, concentrated herbs are the answer, because the concentration is 4 to 6 times of the original herb. Concentrated herbs are taken one step further than the Herbal Extracts: they are freeze-dried to remove the moisture content, thus resulting in a solvent-free product. This powder has all the nutrients in a form that will digest quickly in the blood stream. Concentrated herbs work quickly for pain relief.

Herbal Extracts

BLACK WALNUT EXTRACT — This natural herbal extract contains organic potassium iodine that is very antiseptic and healing. It has been used for syphilis, diphtheria, worms of all types, boils, eczema, itch and ringworm.

CAPSICUM EXTRACT — Can be rubbed on toothaches, inflammation and swellings. Excellent for shock and internal and external bleeding. For the pain of arthritis, rub on the inflammed joints and wrap a flannel cloth for the night.

CATNIP AND FENNEL EXTRACT — Good for stomach cramps, upset stomach, gas, excessive acid in stomach and intestinal tract, fevers, nervous headache and restlessness. A very good extract for colic in infants.

GARLIC OIL — Nature's antibiotic. It is useful for high blood pressure, and for respiratory infections. It has been used for earaches. It is effective in stopping intestinal infections.

GINSENG EXTRACT — Excellent for senility, energy, fatigue and memory. The extract is assimilated into the system faster. It stimulates the system to overcome stress and fatigue. It is useful when recovering from sickness.

GOLDEN SEAL ROOT EXTRACT — It is a powerful tonic which effectively tones mucous membranes and all other tissues it contacts (aids in digestion, improves appetite). It is a remedy for liver congestion and catarrh of the bladder. Excellent for external use.

HAWTHORN BERRY EXTRACT — An excellent remedy for all heart conditions and high and low blood pressure. It helps strengthen the heart muscle. It is effective against insomnia. It is also good for circulation and emotional stress. There are no side effects.

LOBELIA — Lobelia is a general corrector of obstruction of the whole system. It has an influence on the whole system. It is a relaxant and a counter irritant. It can be used with garlic oil for earaches. For teething infants, rub lobelia extract on the swollen gums. For mucus and spasmodic congestion, use by rubbing into the neck, chest and between the shoulders. It is used in water for children.

MULLEIN OIL — This herb is valuable in relieving pain quickly. It is used to relieve pain and irritation of hemorrhoids by applying mullein oil directly onto the affected area. It has been used in relieving the pain of ear infections.

MYRRH EXTRACT — It is an excellent tonic for infected mucous surfaces (gum, throat, ulcers, etc.) and makes a good skin conditioner. It is a good antiseptic, disinfectant and stimulant to open sores and ulcers. It accelerates the healing action and lessens the possibility of inflammation. It increases the circulation and quickens the heart action.

YUCCA EXTRACT — This herb has been used as a food supplement for various forms of arthritis. It helps relieve swellings, pain and stiffness.

COMBINATION NO I EXTRACT — Chickweed, Black Cohosh, Golden Seal, Lobelia, Skullcap, Brigham Tea, Licorice. This herbal extract is useful to help fight infections, especially for all kinds of ear problems, such as ear infections, built up ear wax, ear itching, it has also been used for some types of hearing loss. It can also be used for throat infections.

COMBINATION NO II EXTRACT — Valerian, Anise, Lobelia, Brigham Tea, Black Walnut, Licorice, Ginger. Excellent for nervous disorder and emergencies. It is used as an antispasmodic herbal combination. It has been used for convulsions, high fevers, and any condition to settle the system.

COMBINATION NO III EXTRACT — Dong Quai, Royal Jelly. This herbal extract is useful for skin problems relating to hormone imbalance in females, such as age spots. It can be rubbed on tight muscles to loosen them. It is known for its benefits for female problems.

Common Poultices

BAYBERRY — Can be applied on skin for cancerous and ulcerated sores. It is a strong cleanser and healer.

CATNIP — Reduces swellings, especially good for under the eyes. Culpepper mentions catnip for hemorrhoids, applied topically.

CLAY — Excellent healing agent. Good for skin problems such as eczema. Swollen liver can be helped with clay packs. It is suggested that clay should be taken internally a few days before using as a pack on the body. It can be used for boils, carbuncles and tumors.

COMFREY — An excellent wound-healer and bone-knitter. Can be applied externally for burns, sprains and wounds. It has been used as a hot poultice in helping ease the pain from bursitis.

GINGER — Add powdered ginger to boiling water. Soak a cloth in ginger water, and apply to help relieve pain, or to bring blood to surface in congested areas. Ginger baths, and soaking the feet will help reduce pain.

HOPS — A poultice soothes inflammations and boils and helps reduce the pain of toothache. The Lupulon and Humulon properties help to prevent infections.

MULLEIN — Used for swollen lymph glands and lymph congestion by using 1 part lobelia and 3 parts mullein.

ONION — Used for boils, ears, infections, sore throats, and sores. When using as a poultice, chop and heat the onions.

PLANTAIN — This is a valuable first-aid remedy. Apply mashed or crushed herb on a cut, swollen sore or running sore. Put on finger for whitlow. Secure with clean bandage, disgard pulp, replace as needed.

POTATO — Good for infections, tumors and warts. Use by grating raw potato and add ginger (to stimulate the action of the potato).

SLIPPERY ELM — Excellent for abcesses, bites, blood poison, boils, and stings. Use by combining 1 part lobelia and 2 parts slippery elm. Slippery elm is used as a jelling agent for poultices. It is excellent mixed with other herbs.

WHITE OAK BARK — Use for hemorrhoids and varicose veins.

YARROW — This is a good poultice for wounds, and inflammations. It has been used to reduce swellings and ease earaches. The poultice will also soothe bruises and abrasions. For nosebleeds, the leaves are steeped in water and then placed in the nostrils. Also useful for nicks and cuts. Has anti-inflammatory properties, can be applied as a tea to sore nipples in nursing mothers. It can be used as a wash for eczema, rashes, and poison ivy.

Natural Antiseptics

BLACK WALNUT — external and internal antiseptic, good for internal parasites, infection and tonsillitis.

CABBAGE LEAVES — contains rapine, an antibiotic. The warm leaves placed on the ulcerated sore will draw out the pus on some sores.

CARROTS — mashed and boiled and applied to a sore have helped in drawing out pus and healing the area. It is said to be a strong antiseptic.

CLOVE — the oil is a strong germicide. It is used for toothaches, and pains as well as nausea and vomiting.

CYANI FLOWERS — contains important glycosides which have strong antiseptic properties. This herb has been used in an eyewash. Its antigermicidal and antibacterial properties have been used as an effective antidote against snake venom and scorpion poisons.

FALSE UNICORN — contains chamaelirin, a strong antiseptic. Helps ease evacuation of tapeworms and worms in the intestinal tract. It creates a healthful pure environment in the body.

GARLIC — is a powerful antibacterial agent. It contains Allicin. The powder on wounds is good for the healing process. Garlic oil is useful for ear infections.

GOLDEN SEAL — contains antibiotic berberine which is used for mouth and gum problems. It is also used for worms and infection.

LEMONS — a natural antiseptic — destroys harmful bacteria. Helps fade freckles.

MYRRH — has sensational antiseptic properties, contains gums, essential oils, resin and other bitter compounds. Good for uterus and vaginal infections and dysentery. It is also used for serious peridontal diseases. Laboratory tests have proven this to be one of the finest antibacterial and anti-viral agents.

THYME — contains antiseptic properties called thymol. Use small amounts for dressing wounds. When it is crushed and added to boiling water, and then steeped and strained, it can be used for sprains and bruises.

QUEEN OF THE MEADOW — used as an antiseptic to treat diseases of the uterus and cancer of the womb.

SECTION VI

Single Herbs

AGRIMONY   (ag′-ra-mō-nē)
(*Agrimonia eupatoria*)
Parts used: The Herb

Agrimony strengthens the whole system, but it works chiefly on the liver. The astringent properties contract and harden tissue. It is absorbed in the system to strengthen and tone the muscles of the body and is therefore a useful tonic. It affects the cells of the kidneys, allowing fluids to pass more readily through the kidneys, so it is a useful diuretic. The astringent qualities of Agrimony help draw thorns and splinters from the skin. It has been recommended to help acidity and gastric ulcers, because it is a good, safe stomach tonic which helps in the assimilation of food.

Agrimony contains vitamins B₃, K, iron and niacin.

DIARRHEA
Fevers
Gallbladder
GASTRIC DISORDERS
Hemorrhoids
INTESTINES
JAUNDICE
KIDNEY STONES

LIVER DISORDERS
Rheumatism
Skin diseases
Sore throat
Splinters
Sprains
Wounds, external

ALFALFA   (ăl-făl'-fa)
(Medicago sativa)
Parts used: Leaves and Flowers

Alfalfa contains health building properties. It helps assimilate protein, calcium and other nutrients. It is beneficial for all ailments because of its vitality and nutrient properties. And the contents are also balanced for complete absorption. Alfalfa contains chlorophyll. It is a body cleanser, infection fighter and natural deodorizer. It breaks down poisonous carbon dioxide and it is the richest land source of trace minerals. It is a very good spring tonic, it eliminates retained water, and relieves urinary and bowel problems. It helps in treating recuperative cases of narcotic and alcohol addiction. The enzymes help to neutralize cancer in the system.

Alfalfa contains a very rich supply of vitamins A, K, and D. It is also high in calcium and contains phosphorus, iron, potassium and eight essential enzymes. It is rich in trace minerals.

Alcoholism	FATIGUE, (MENTAL AND
Allergies	PHYSICAL)
ANEMIA	Fever reducer
Appendicitis, chronic	Gout
APPETITE STIMULANT	HEMORRHAGES
ARTHRITIS	High blood pressure
BLOOD PURIFIER	Jaundice
Body building	KIDNEY CLEANSER
Bowel problems	Lactation (quantity and
Bursitis	quality of milk)
Cancer	NAUSEA
Cholesterol reducer	Nosebleeds
Cramps	PITUITARY PROBLEMS
DIABETES	Teeth
Digestion	TONIC
Diuretic (mild)	ULCERS, PEPTIC
	Urinary problems

ALOE VERA (ăl'-ō va'-ră)
(Aloe vera)
Parts used: Leaves

Aloe Vera is known as the first aid plant. It cleans, soothes and heals. It also contains antibiotic properties. It shouldn't be taken as a laxative during pregnancy. It contains properties which promote the removal of dead skin and stimulates the normal growth of living cells and which can stop pain and reduce the chance of infection and scarring while helping the healing process.

This is one plant every household should have. It is one of the easiest plants to grow indoors. It is valuable to burning, itching, minor cuts and first and second degree thermal burns. The fresh juice from the leaves heals wounds by preventing or drawing out infections. Aloe Vera helps to heal internal tissues damaged by radiation exposure such as x-rays and radiation.

Aloe Vera contains calcium, potassium, sodium, manganese, magnesium, iron, lecithin, and zinc.

Abrasions
Acne
Anemia
BURNS
Constipation
DEODORANT
DIGESTION
Heartburn
HEMORRHOIDS
INSECT BITES
Leg ulcers
Poison ivy and oak

Psoriasis
RADIATION BURNS
Ringworm
SCALDS
SCAR TISSUE
Sores
Sunburn
Tapeworm
Tuberculosis
Wrinkling of skin
Ulcered sores
Ulcers, peptic

AMARANTH   (am'-a-ranth)
(Amaranthus spp.)
Parts used: Leaves and Flowers

Amaranth is used for gastroenteritis or stomach flu. It lessens irritability of the tissues. Topical application can reduce tissue swelling. The saponine content in Amaranth can be used to produce a lather. It has been used for bandages for medical treatments. A strong decoction can be used as a vermifuge (remove worms and other parasites from the digestive tract). Amaranth is a vitamin-packed herb and was used by the Indians as a survival food. The mature seeds were eaten raw or mixed with corn meal or added to soups. The leaves were used in place of spinach.

Amaranth is very high in iron and vitamin C. It is also high in calcium and protein and contains phosphorus, potassium, thiamine, riboflavin and niacin.

Canker sores	NOSE BLEEDS
DIARRHEA	Ulcers (stomach and mouth)
DYSENTERY	Worms
Gums, bleeding	Wounds
MENSTRUATION, EXCESSIVE	

ANGELICA   (an-jel'-i-ka)
(Angelica atropurpurea)
Parts used: Root

Angelica is very helpful in colic and digestive problems. It is considered a tonic to improve well being and mental harmony. There is a caution for diabetics, because it increases sugar in the blood. It is also an emmenagogue, so it should not be used by pregnant women. Culpepper said the juice of the plant had been used in the eyes and ears to help dimness of sight and deafness. It is also used for toothaches. It cleans wounds and helps them to heal quickly, and is useful in all sorts of stomach and intestinal difficulties, including ulcers and vomiting with stomach cramps. It can be used for intermittent fever, nervous headache, colic, and general weakness.

Angelica contains vitamin E, calcium, and some species of this plant contain vitamin B_{12}, which is rare in vegetation.

APPETITE STIMULANT	GAS
Arthritis	HEARTBURN
BRONCHIAL PROBLEMS	Inflammation
Backaches	Lung problems
COLDS	Menstrual disorders
COLIC	Prostate problems
COUGHS	RHEUMATISM
Digestive problems	Sores
Ears (drops for deafness)	Stomach cramps
EPIDEMICS	TONIC
EXHAUSTION	Toothaches
Fevers	

ANISE (án-as)
(Pimpinella anisum)
Parts used: Oil and Seeds

Anise is helpful in removing excess mucus and in preventing the possible formation of catarrh along the alimentary canal. It is said by some herbalists that Anise seems high in estrogen content, which tends to stimulate all the glands. Anise is used for loss of appetite, difficulty of digestion, mucus obstruction in coughs and whooping cough. It is used as a stimulant for vital organs of the body such as heart, liver, lungs and brain. It is one of the best herbs for relieving pains for colic.

Anise contains the B vitamins, choline, calcium, iron, potassium and magnesium.

Appetite stimulant
Breath sweetener
Catarrh
Colds (hard and dry)
COLIC
CONVULSIONS
COUGHS

Epilepsy
GAS
INTESTINAL PURIFIER
MUCUS
Nausea
Nervousness
Pneumonia

BARBERRY (bär'-bĕr'-ē)
(Berberis vulgaris)
Parts used: Bark

Barberry contains the antiseptic properties which make it useful as a gargle and mouthwash. It is called one of the best medicinal herb plants of the west. Barberry is used in fevers and inflammatory conditions. Its influence upon the liver is so effective that the bile will flow more freely, which is important in almost all liver problems, especially jaundice. It also helps remove morbid matter from the stomach and bowels. It dilates the blood vessels, therefore it is good for high blood pressure.

Barberry is high in vitamin C. It contains iron, manganese, and phosphorus.

Arthritis
Blood pressure, (lowers)
BLOOD PURIFIER
Constipation
DIARRHEA
Dysentery
Dyspepsia
Fevers
Gall Bladder
Gum diseases

Hemorrhages
INDIGESTION
JAUNDICE
Laxative
LIVER PROBLEMS
Pyorrhea
Spleen problems
THROAT (SORE)
Ulcers

BARLEY JUICE POWDER

Barley juice powder is produced from the juice of young barley leaves. It is essentially the same as the fresh juice. It contains concentrated nutrients, live enzymes, chlorophyll, proteins, vitamins and minerals. It contains anti-viral properties. It is a great booster for the immune system. It has a cleansing effect on the cells, normalizes metabolism and neutralizes heavy metals like mercury.

'It helps to lower cholesterol while purifying the blood. It will help relieve constipation. It helps balance body chemistry, and is an excellent cell detoxifier. It purifies and builds up the blood with its high iron content. It helps digestion, therefore strengthening the whole body.

It is rich in calcium, iron, vitamin C and bioflavoinoids. It contains B1 and B12. It contains Superoxide dismutase (SOD). It is rich in magnesium and potassium.

Acne	Herpes
Aids	Infections
Allergies	Kidney problems
ANEMIA	Leprosy
ARTHRITIS	Liver problems
BLOOD PURIFIER	Lung problems
BOILS	METAL POISONING
Bronchitis	Psoriasis
Candida Albicans	Skin diseases
CANCER	Syphilis
Eczema	Tuberculosis
Hay fever	Ulcers

BASIL   (băz-el)
(Ocimum basilicum)
Parts used: Leaves

Basil has been effectively used as a stimulant in cases of collapse. It also has strong antibacterial and antispasmodic properties, making it useful for whooping cough and in drawing out poisons when applied to wasp and hornet stings or venomous bites.
Basil contains vitamins A, D, and B2. Basil contains lots of calcium, phosphorus, iron, and magnesium.

BITES (INSECT, SNAKE)	Kidney problems
Bladder problems	Menstruation (suppressed)
Catarrh (intestinal)	Nausea
Constipation	Nervous conditions
COLDS	Respiratory infections
Cramps (stomach)	Rheumatism
Fevers	Vomiting (excessive)
Flu	WHOOPING COUGH
HEADACHES	Worms
INDIGESTION	

BAYBERRY   (bā'-běr'-ē)
(Myrica cerifera)
Parts used: Bark

Bayberry can be useful in warding off colds at the first signs, especially when taken along with Capsicum. It is also used as a gargle for tonsillitis and sore throat. It is beneficial in rejuvenation of the adrenal glands, cleansing the blood stream, washing out wastes in veins and arteries and ridding the system of poisonous wastes. In India, the powdered root bark of Bayberry has been combined with Ginger to successfully combat the deadly effects of cholera. Bayberry has long been used as

a tonic, stimulating the system to help raise vitality and resistance to disease and at the same time to aid digestion, nutrition and building the blood.
Bayberry contains a high amount of Vitamin C.

Bleeding	JAUNDICE
Catarrh	Liver problems
CHOLERA	MENSTRUAL BLEEDING,
Colitis (mucus in)	EXCESSIVE
DIARRHEA	SCROFULA
DYSENTERY	Sluggishness
Dyspepsia	Scurvy
GLANDS	Throat, sore and ulcerated
GOITER	Ulcers
Gums, bleeding	UTERINE HEMORRHAGE
INDIGESTION	Uterus, prolapsed

BEE POLLEN   (bē pol'-ăn)
Parts used: Bee Pollen

Bee pollen is high in aspartic acid, an amino acid that is able to stimulate the glands to promote a feeling of physical rejuvenation. It promotes youthful feeling, builds resistance to diseases, helps to boost healing powers and provides the body with energy.

Studies have found that it has a healing effect where there is pernicious anemia and disturbances of the intestinal system such as colitis, and chronic constipation. Bee Pollen slows down the aging process, for it has helped the emotional well-being of aging people. It also helps the hormonal system. Bee Pollen mixed with honey is used in Russia for treating hypertension, nervous and endocrine system complaints. It normalizes the activity of the intestines (in cases of colitis or chronic constipation), improves the appetite, and increases fitness for work. Some people could be allergic to Bee Pollen and caution should be used if itching, dizziness, or difficulty in swallowing occurs after taking it. Always start out with small doses.

Bee Pollen contains 35% protein, about half of which is in the form of free amino acids, which are essential to life and can be immediately assimilated by the body. It is high in B-complex vitamins, and also vitamins A, C, D, and E. It is said to contain every substance needed to maintain life. It is called a complete food. Bee Pollen also contains Lecithin.

ALLERGIES	HAY FEVER
Asthma	Hypoglycemia
Blood pressure (lowers)	Indigestion
Cancer	Liver diseases
Depression	LONGEVITY
Endurance	Prostate disorders
ENERGY	Vitality
EXHAUSTION	

BILBERRY   (bil' ber"ry)
(Vaccinium myrtillus)
Parts used: Fruit

Bilberry is an old remedy, rediscovered. Research has found its properties to be beneficial for the eyes. It strengthens the capillaries, the small veins that surround the eyes. It improves circulation and feeds the capillaries by altering the ability of fluids and nourishment to pass through.

Bilberry can benefit all capillaries, veins and arteries, thus improving circulation to the feet, hands, brain, and heart. It has properties to strengthen coronary arteries, varicose veins and help in reducing atherosclerosis or the obstruction of arteries by plaque deposits. Blood clots can be reduced, by the thinning properties of Bilberry. It inhibits blood platelets sticking together.

It is considered a beneficial herb to be used in preventing cataracts, along with vitamin E, and other supplements that supply oxygen to the blood. It has the ability to protect the eyes against damage created by diabetes.

Bilberry is rich in bioflavonoids. It is also rich in manganese, phosphorus, iron and zinc. It contains moderate amounts of magnesium, potassium and selenium. It contains trace amounts of calcium, sodium and silicon.

Blood thinner
BLOOD VESSELS
COLD HANDS & FEET
Diarrhea
Dropsy
Immune system
Kidney problems

Light sensitive
NIGHT BLINDNESS
Raynaud's Disease
Scurvy
Typhoid epidemics
VARICOSE VEINS

BIRCH (būrch)
(Betula alba)
Parts used: Bark and Leaves

Birch contains natural properties for cleansing the blood. The dry distillation of the bark produces the "birch oil" which is used in cases of certain skin complaints. Birch bark also contains a glycoside which decomposes to give methyl salicylate. It is used as a remedy for rheumatism both in Canada and the United States. A decoction of the leaves is recommended for baldness. For insomnia, a decoction is used as a mild sedative. The powder of Birch can be used to brush teeth.

Birch is high in natural fluoride. It contains vitamins A, C, E, and B_1 and B_2 of the complex vitamins, but also contains calcium, chlorine, copper, iron, magnesium, phosphorus, potassium, sodium, and silicon.

BLADDER   ECZEMA, EXTERNAL
Bleeding gums   Fevers
BLOOD CLEANSER   Gout
Cankers   Kidneys
Cholera   Pyorrhea
Diarrhea   Urinary tract
Dysentery   Worms (expels)
Dropsy

BISTORT   (bis'-tòrt)
(Polygonum bistorta)
Parts used: Root

Bistort is one of the strongest astringents in the herb kingdom with antiseptic properties. It is a member of the buckwheat
family and can therefore be used as an emergency food. The
root contains starch, and in times of famine it was dried and
ground up for use as flour. Bistort is useful in all bleeding
internally and externally. The powdered Bistort can be applied
to wounds, and is good for infectious diseases, and driving them
out by sweating. It is used as a decoction for mouthwash, gum
problems, and mouth inflammations. Externally, it is used as a
wash for sores and hemorrhages.

Bistort contains vitamin A, is rich in vitamin C, and
contains some B-complex vitamin.

BLEEDING, external and   Jaundice
   internal   Measles
Bowels   Menstruation (regulation of)
Canker sores   MOUTHWASH
CHOLERA   Mucus
CUTS   Plague
Diabetes   Small Pox
DIARRHEA   Tonic, spring
DYSENTERY   Worms (expels)
GUMS
HEMORRHOIDS

BLACKBERRY   (blăk-bēr'-ē)
(Rubus fructicosus)
Parts used: Leaves and Root Bark

Blackberry, when used as a tea, can dry up sinus drainage. An infusion of the unripe berries is highly esteemed for curing vomiting and loose bowels. The root contains astringent properties. The young shoots are credited with fastening loose teeth in the gums. The Indians used the root tea with success for dysentery. The Chinese believe the fruit increases the "yin principle", in addition to giving vigor to the whole body.
Blackberry contains vitamins A and C. It also contains iron, calcium, riboflavin, niacin and some thiamine.

Anemia	Gargle
BLEEDING	Genital irritations
Boils	Gums, bleeding
Blackheads	Menstruation, excessive
CHOLERA	Mouth irritations
DIARRHEA (CHILDREN)	Peristalsis, weak
Dropsy	Rheumatism
DYSENTERY	SINUS DRAINAGE
Eye wash	Sores
Female problems	Stomach, upset
Fevers	VOMITING

BLACK COHOSH   (blăk kō'-häsh)
(Cimicifuga racemosa)
Parts used: Root

Black Cohosh is used as a tonic for the central nervous system. It is an excellent, safe sedative. It contains natural estrogen, the female hormone. It helps in hot flashes, contracts the uterus and increases menstrual flow when sluggish. It also loosens and expels mucus of the bronchial tubes and stimulates the secretions of the liver, kidneys and lymphs. A poultice can be used for all kinds of inflammation. A syrup can be used for coughs. It has the ability to neutralize poisons in the bloodstream, and helps uric acid and toxic wastes in the body. It equalizes blood circulation.

Black Cohosh contains effective amounts of calcium, potassium, magnesium, and iron. It contains some vitamin A, inositol, pantothenic acid, silicon, and phosphorus.

Arthritis	Insomnia
ASTHMA	Kidney problems
Bites, insect and snake	Liver problems
BRONCHITIS, CHRONIC	Lumbago
and acute	LUNGS
Childbirth	MENOPAUSE
Cholera	MENSTRUAL PROBLEMS
Convulsions	Nervous disorders
Coughs	Neuralgia
Cramps	Pain
EPILEPSY	Rheumatism
Headaches	Skin problems
Heart stimulant	Smallpox
HIGH BLOOD PRESSURE	ST. VITUS DANCE
HORMONE BALANCE	TUBERCULOSIS
Hot flashes	Uterine problems
Hysteria	WHOOPING COUGH

BLACK WALNUT   (blăk wōl'-nūt)
(Juglans nigra)
Parts used: Hulls and Leaves

Black Walnut oxygenates the blood to kill parasites. It is used to help balance sugar levels. It also is able to burn up excessive toxins and fatty materials.

The extract is very useful for poison oak, ringworm and skin problems.

The brown stain found in the green husk contains organic **iodine** which has antiseptic and healing properties.

Black walnut is used for restoring tooth enamel. It contains constituents which have been found to be a protective antidote for electrical shock.

Black Walnut is rich in vitamin B₁₅ and manganese. It contains magnesium, silica, protein, calcium, phosphorus, iron and potassium.

Abscesses
Acne
Antiperspirant
ANTISEPTIC, EXTERNAL
Boils
Cancer
Carbuncles
Colitis
Diphtheria
Eczema
Eye diseases
Fevers
Gargle
Hemorrhoids
Infections
LACTATION, STOPS
Liver
Lupus
Mouthsores
PARASITES, INTERNAL
Piles, bleeding
Poison Ivy
RASHES, SKIN
RINGWORM
Scrofula
Tonsillitus
Tuberculosis
Tumors
Ulcers, internal
Uterus, prolapsed
Varicose veins
WORMS
Wounds

BLESSED THISTLE   (blĕs'-ĭd thĭs'-al)
(Cnicus benedictus)
Parts used: The Herb

Blessed Thistle has a long history as a digestive and general tonic. It is useful for headaches in menopause problems. It is an excellent tonic for stomach and heart, aids circulation and helps all liver problems. It increases mothers' milk, and strengthens the memory by bringing oxygen to the brain. It helps control fevers, helps with cramps and other female problems, and also helps in balancing hormones. The Quinault Indians used the whole plant, steeped to create a birth-control medicine. It also has been used for treating internal cancer.

Blessed Thistle contains the B-complex vitamin, manganese, calcium, iron, phosphorus, and potassium.

Arthritis	HORMONES (BALANCES)
Birth control	Jaundice
BLOOD CIRCULATION	Kidneys
BLOOD PURIFIER	LACTATION
Cancer	Leucorrhea
Constipation	LIVER AILMENTS
Cramps	LUNGS (STRENGTHENS)
DIGESTION	Memory (strengthens)
Dropsy	MENSTRUAL PROBLEMS
Fevers	Respiratory infection
GALL BLADDER	Senility
Gas	Spleen
HEADACHES	Worms
HEART (STRENGTHENS)	

BLUE COHOSH   (bloo kō'-häsh)
(Caulophyllum thalictroides)
Parts used: Root

Blue Cohosh contains antibacterial properties and complementary properties for the nerves. It has a strong antispasmodic effect on the whole system. It can relieve muscle cramps, spasms, and is also helpful in relieving painful menstruation. It helps to stretch the neck of the uterus so delivery is easier. If Black Cohosh is given hours previous to delivery, it is said to be reliable and less dangerous where cases of labor is slow and very painful. Because of the emmenagogue properties, it should not be used by pregnant women except the last month. Blue Cohosh should be used in combination with other herbs, such as Black Cohosh.

Blue Cohosh contains vitamins E and B-complex. It also contains calcium, magnesium, phosphorus and potassium.

Ague	Colic
Bladder infection	Convulsions

CRAMPS	Menstruation (regulation of)
Diabetes	NERVES
Dropsy	Neuralgia
EPILEPSY	Pregnancy disorders
Fits	Spasms
High blood pressure	UTERINE, (CHRONIC
LABOR (INDUCES)	PROBLEMS)
Leucorrhea	Vaginitis

BLUE VERVAIN (bloo ver'-vān)
(Verbena hastata)
Parts used: The Herb

Blue Vervain is used as a natural tranquilizer, and as an antiperiodic for all nervous problems. It has the ability to promote sweating and relaxation, allay fevers, stomach settling and producing an overall feeling of well being. Blue Vervain is one of the best herbs to use to help alleviate the onset of a virus cold, especially with upper respiratory inflammation. It will expel phlegm from the throat and chest. It is useful in menstrual problems.

Blue Vervain contains vitamin C and some vitamin E. It also contains calcium and manganese.

Ague	Female problems
ASTHMA	FEVERS
BLADDER	Gallstones
BOWELS	Headaches
BRONCHITIS	INSOMNIA
Catarrh	Kidney problems
COLDS	Menstrual problems
COLON	Mucus
CONSUMPTION	Nerves
Congestion, throat and chest	Pneumonia
CONVULSIONS	Skin diseases
COUGHS	Sores
Diarrhea	Spleen
Dysentery	STOMACH (SETTLES)
Earaches	WORMS
Epilepsy	

BONESET   (bōn'-set)
(Eupatorium perfoliatum)
Parts used: The Herb

Boneset is excellent for influenza. Dr. Shook says that he has never known this herb to fail in overcoming influenza.

Boneset tea was one of the most common home remedies in the last century. The Indians used it to reduce fever, to relieve body pain and for colds. It was given the name of "Break-bone fever" because of the pain influenza caused that felt like breaking bones. It is a mild tonic and very useful in the indigestion of old people.

Boneset contains vitamin C, calcium, some PABA, and also contains magnesium and potassium.

Bronchitis	Mumps
Catarrh	Rheumatism, muscular
CHILLS	Rocky Mountain Spotted
COLDS	Fever
FEVER PREVENTION	Scarlet Fever
FEVERS (ALL KINDS)	Throat (sore)
FLU	Tonic
Jaundice	TYPHOID FEVER
Liver disorders	Worms
Malaria	YELLOW FEVER
Measles	

BORAGE   (bȯr'-ij)
(Borago officinalis)
Parts used: Leaves

Borage is especially soothing in bronchitis and for the digestive system. It promotes the activity of the kidneys to dispose of feverish catarrh. Borage has a stimulating effect to the adrenal glands. It acts on the kidneys to dispose of feverish catarrh. It is said to be good in restoring vitality during recovery from illness. It is soothing to the mucous membranes of the mouth and throat. The tea can be used as an eyewash for sore eyes, and it has been used to increase mother's milk. Borage contains potassium and calcium.

Bladder	Jaundice
Blood purifier	Insomia preventative
BRONCHITIS	LACTATION
CATARRH (CHRONIC)	Nerves (calms)
Colds, fever	Pleurisy
Digestion	RASHES
EYES (INFLAMMATION)	RINGWORM
HEART (STRENGTHENS)	

BUCHU   (bōō'-koō)
(Barosma betulina)
Parts used: Leaves

Buchu has a healing influence on all chronic complaints of the genito-urinary tract. One of the best herbs of the urinary organs, Buchu absorbs excessive uric acid, reducing bladder irritations and "scalding urine." Buchu increases the quantity of urinic fluids and solids, and at the same time it acts as a tonic and astringent and disinfectant to the mucous membranes. It is said to be useful for the first stages of diabetes.

It has been combined with Uva Ursi for treatment of water retention and urinary tract infections. When taken warm, it is used in treatment of enlargement of the prostate gland and irritation of the membrane of the urethra.

Bed wetting	KIDNEY PROBLEMS
BLADDER CATARRH	NEPHRITIS
Cystitis	PROSTATE PROBLEMS
Diabetes (first stages)	Rheumatism
Dropsy	URETHRITIS
Gallstones	Yeast infections

BUCKTHORN   (bŭk'-thôrn')
(Rhamnus frangula)
Parts used: Bark and Berries

Buckthorn has a stimulating effect on the bile. It does not gripe, and it has a calming effect on the gastrointestinal tract, without being habit forming. It can be used for longer periods without discomfort. If taken hot, it will produce perspiration and lowers fevers. The ointment of the herb helps provide relief from itching. The leaves bruised and applied to the wound will stop bleeding.

Appendicitis	Hemorrhoids
BLEEDING	Itching
BOWELS	LEAD POISONING
CONSTIPATION	LIVER
(CHRONIC)	Parasites
Dropsy	Rheumatism
FEVERS	Skin diseases
GALLSTONES	Warts, external
Gout	Worms

BUGLEWEED   (byü'-gel-wēd)
(Lycopus virginicus)
Parts used: The Herb

Bugleweed is very useful on painful areas of the body. It is able to bring some relief to where the pain is located. It contains compounds that contract tissues of the mucous membrane and reduces fluid discharges. It is an herb that increases the appetite, but is also used for enlargement of the thyroid gland. Its action resembles that of digitalis, lowering the pulse and lessening its frequency. It helps irritations of coughs, and equalizes circulation. It is termed one of the mildest and best narcotics in the world.

Bleeding	MENSTRUATION,
COUGHS	EXCESS
Colds	NERVES
Diabetes	Nosebleeds
Diarrhea	PAIN
Fevers	Sores
Hemorrhages, pulmonary	Tuberculosis
INDIGESTION, NERVOUS	Ulcers

BURDOCK (bûr'-dŏk')
(Arctium lappa)
Parts used: Root

Burdock is one of the best blood purifiers, it can reduce swelling around joints and helps rid calcification deposits, for it promotes kidney function to help clear the blood of harmful acids. Burdock contains anywhere from 27 to 45% inulin, a form of starch, which is the source of most of its curative powers. Inulin is a substance that is important in the metabolism of carbohydrates. In Europe it is used as a remedy for prolapsed and displaced uterus. Burdock, when mixed with Sassafras and made into a tea, is said to release a strong oil that is soothing to the hypothalamus. It also aids the pituitary gland in releasing an ample supply of protein to help adjust hormone balance in the body. It is said that a poorly nourished pituitary gland is sometimes responsible for overweight.

Burdock contains a lot of vitamin C and iron. It contains 12% protein, 70% carbohydrate, some vitamin A, P, and B-complex, vitamin E, PABA, and small amounts of sulphur, silicon, copper, iodine and zinc.

Acne	Bronchitis
Allergies	Canker sores
ARTHRITIS	Cancer
Asthma	Dandruff
BLOOD PURIFIER	ECZEMA
Boils	Fevers

GOUT
Hay ·fever
Infections
KIDNEY PROBLEMS
Leprosy
Liver problems
Lumbago

LUNGS
Nervousness
RHEUMATISM
SKIN DISEASES
Uterus, prolapsed
Wounds

BUTCHER'S BROOM (butch' eris broom)
(Ruscus aculeatus)
Parts used: Rhizomes

Butcher's Broom was used centuries ago. Research on this herb revealed that it has a strengthening effect on the vessel-walls as well as containing anti-inflammatory properties. It has a constricting action on the veins, making it effective when used on patients with post-operative tendency toward circulatory problems.

Butcher's Broom has been beneficial for improving periferal circulation, to prevent post-operative thrombosis, varicose veins, phlebitis, hemorrhoids and circulatory problems.

It increases circulation to the brain, legs and arms. It has a diuretic effect, and causes the constriction of blood vessels. It will help prevent atherosclerosis and lower the level of cholesterol. Circulatory problems being the number one killer in the United States, it would be wise to consider Butcher's Broom.

ATHEROSCLEROSIS
Brain (circulation)
Circulation (increases)
Dropsy
Headaches
HEMORRHOIDS
Jaundice

Leg cramps
Menstrual problems
Phlebitis (vein
   inflammation)
THROMBOSIS (BLOOD
   CLOTTING)
VARICOSE VEINS

CAPSICUM or CAYENNE (kăp'-sĭ-kam)
(Capsicum frutescens)
Parts used: Fruit

Capsicum is said to be unequalled for warding off diseases and equalizing blood circulation. It is called a "Supreme and harmless internal disinfectant." It increases the heart action but not the blood pressure. It is said to prevent strokes and heart attacks. It is used for hemorrhaging external and internal.

Capsicum increases the power of all other herbs, helps in digestion when taken with meals and promotes all the secreting organs. It is a natural stimulant for diarrhea and dysentery.

This herb is a very important one when you want quick action for the flu and colds for its stimulating action.

It has the ability to rebuild tissue in the stomach and heals stomach and intestinal ulcers. It is known as the purest and best stimulant in the herb kingdom. It is said to be a catalyst, carrying all other herbs quickly to the part of the body where it is most needed, and increases their effectiveness.

Capsicum is high in Vitamins A, C, iron and calcium. It has Vitamin G, Magnesium, Phosphorus, and Sulphur. It has some B-complex, and is rich in Potassium.

Ague
ARTHRITIS
BLEEDING
Blood cleanser
BLOOD PRESSURE
    EQUALIZER
Bronchitis
Bruises
Burns
Congestion
Chills
CIRCULATION
DIABETES
Eyes
Fatigue
Fevers
Gas
HEART
HIGH BLOOD PRESSURE
Infection
Jaundice
KIDNEY PROBLEMS

Lockjaw
Lung problems
Mucus
Pancreas
Pyorrhea
RHEUMATISM
Shock
Sprains, external

STROKES
Sunburns
Throat, sore
TUMORS
ULCERS
Varicose veins
Wounds

CARAWAY   (kar'-a-wā)
(Carum carvi)
Parts used: Seeds

Caraway is a powerful antiseptic which is especially useful in relieving toothaches. It is similar to Anise. The two oils are highly recommended for the same purposes. Caraway is very useful when mixed with other herbs, for it helps to correct or modify the action of purgatives such as Mandrake and Culver's Root. When applied locally to the skin, it acts as an anesthetic. It helps prevent fermentation in the stomach, and to help settle the stomach after taking nauseous medicines. It is useful for all stomach problems, encourages menstruation and the flow of milk, is good for uterine cramps, mucus in the lungs and intestinal gas in infants.

Caraway contains the B-complex vitamin. It is high in calcium and potassium, but also contains smaller amounts of magnesium, lead,.silicon, zinc, some iodine, copper, cobalt, and iron.

APPETITE STIMULANT
Colds
COLIC
CRAMPS, UTERINE
DIGESTION (ACIDS)
Female problems
GAS

Lactation
Mucus in lungs
Menstruation promotor
SPASM
Stomach (settles)
Toothaches

CASCARA SAGRADA (kăs-kăr'-a sa-grī-da)
(Rhamnus purshiana)
Parts used: Bark

Cascara Sagrada is a bark rich in hormone-like oils which promote peristaltic action in the intestinal canal. It is one of the best herbs to use for chronic constipation and is said to not be habit-forming. It increases the secretions of the stomach, liver, and pancreas and exerts a remarkable action in torpor of the colon in constipation.

It has been effective to the gall ducts, and in helping the body rid itself of gallstones.

Cascara is very valuable whenever there are hemorrhoids because of poor bowel function.

It helps in painless evacuations and, after extended usage, the bowels will function naturally and regularly from its tonic effects. It also has a stimulating tonic effect to all nerves that it comes in contact with. It is very cleansing to the colon and helps rebuild its functions.

Cascara Sagrada contains B-Complex, calcium, potassium, manganese, traces of tin, lead, strontium and aluminum.

Catarrh
COLON
CONSTIPATION
Coughs
Croup
Digestion
Dyspepsia
GALL BLADDER
Gallstones
Gout
Hemorrhoids

High blood pressure
Indigestion
Insomnia
INTESTINES
Jaundice
LIVER DISORDERS
Nerves
Pituitary
Spleen
Worms

CATNIP   (kăt'-nĭp')
(Nepeta cataria)
Parts used: The Herb

Catnip has been called nature's "Alka-Seltzer." The Indians used it for infant colic, but it also has a sedative effect on
the nervous system. It is useful for many ailments: for all cases
of fevers for its action in inducing sleep and in producing
perspiration without increasing heat in the body. In children it is
said to speedily overcome convulsions. It is also good for
restlessness and colic and as a pain killer, especially for small
children and infants. It has been known to help prevent a cold
when drinking a warm infusion when you notice the first
symptom. It helps in fatigue and improves circulation. It is said
to help to prevent miscarriages and premature births. It helps in
aches and pain due to flu and upset stomach and diarrhea
associated with flu.

Catnip is high in vitamins A and C, and the B-complex
vitamin. It contains magnesium, manganese, phosphorus,
sodium, and has a trace of sulphur.

Anemia	Hiccups
Bronchitis, chronic	Infertility
Circulation (improves)	Insanity
COLDS	Lung congestion
COLIC	Menstruation, suppressed
CONVULSIONS	Miscarriage preventive
Coughs	Morning sickness
Cramps, menstrual	Nicotine withdrawal
Cramps, muscle	NERVES
DIARRHEA	Pain
DIGESTION	Restlessness
Diseases, childhood	Shock
Drug withdrawal	Skin
Fatigue	Sores, external
FEVERS	Spasms
FLU	Stress
GAS	Stomach upset
Headaches, nervous	Vomiting
Hemorrhoids	Worms

CELERY   (sel'-rē)
(Apium graveolens)
Parts used: Root and Seeds

The seeds and stems of Celery have been used in Australia as an acid neutralizer. It should be cooked with milk and eaten freely to neutralize uric acid and other excess acids in the body, thus aiding in the treatment of rheumatism. Celery is useful for headaches when taken as a tea. It produces perspiration and is useful for nervousness. It has a stimulating effect on the kidneys, producing an increased flow of urine.

Celery contains vitamins A, B, and C and has lots of calcium, potassium, phosphorus, sodium, and iron. It also contains smaller amounts of sulphur, silicon, and magnesium.

ARTHRITIS	Liver problems
Bright's disease	LUMBAGO
Catarrah, post-nasal	NERVOUSNESS
Diabetes	Neuralgia
Dropsy	RHEUMATISM
Gout	Urine retention
Headaches	Vomiting
Insomnia	

CENTAURY   (sen'-tor-ē)
(Erythraea centaurium)
Parts used: The Herb

Centaury is useful during a slow convalescence by promoting appetite and strengthening the digestive system. It purifies the blood and is an excellent tonic. It is good in muscular rheumatism and strengthens the bladder of the elderly. This herb helps prevent bed-wetting. It regulates the gall bladder, and is known as a preventive in all periodic febrile diseases, dyspepsia, and recovery from fevers. It has a healing effect on wounds. Centaury acts as a diffusive stimulating tonic to the heart, stomach, liver, generative organs and the nervous system.

Bed wetting	MENSTRUATION
BLOOD PURIFIER	PROMOTOR
DIGESTION PROMOTER	Rheumatism
Eczema	Sores, external
FEVERS	Tonic
High blood pressure	Ulcers
Gall bladder	Worms
Jaundice	Wounds, external
Liver	

CHAMOMILE   (kăm'-a-mīl')
(Anthemis nobilis)
Parts used: Flower

Chamomile is one of the best herbs to keep handy for emergencies, for it is both beneficial and trustworthy. It is a welcome tea for nerves and menstrual cramps. Chamomile helps promote a natural hormone, like thyroxine, which helps rejuvenate the texture of the hair and skin, and also helps in youthful mental alertness. It is a soothing sedative with no harmful effects. It is useful for small babies and children for colds, stomach trouble, colitis, a gargle, and externally for eczema and inflammation. It is one of the best herbs for soothing an upset stomach and colic in babies and inducing sleep. It is recognized by orothodox medical profession as a valuable medicine for the young, especially in France and Spain, where numerous doctors prescribe it.

Chamomile contains a high content of calcium, and magnesium but also has potassium, iron, manganese and zinc. It also contains some vitamin A.

Air pollution	BRONCHITIS
APPETITE STIMULANT	Catarrh
Asthma, (steam inhalant)	Childhood diseases
Bladder problems	Constipation

Colds

Coughs

CRAMPS, MENSTRUAL

Cramps, stomach

Diarrhea

Drug, withdrawal

Earache compress

Eye, sore

FEVERS

Gallstones

Gas

Headaches

HYSTERIA

Indigestion

INSOMNIA

Jaundice

Kidneys

Measles

MENSTRUAL
 SUPPRESSANT

NERVOUSNESS

Pain

Spasms

Stomach upset

Teething

Throat (gargle)

Tumors

Typhoid

Ulcers, peptic

CHAPARRAL (shăp'-a-răl')
(Larrea divaricata)
Parts used: Leaves and Stems

Chaparral has the ability to cleanse deep into the muscles and tissue walls. It is a potent healer to the urethral tract and to lymphatics, tones up the system and rebuilds the tissues. Medical science believes that the process by which Chaparral supports the system works by inhibiting the unwanted rapid growth, via the vital respiratory process throughout the whole system. It is a strong antioxidant, anti-tumor agent, pain-killer, and antiseptic. It is one of the best herbal antibiotics. Chaparral has been said to be able to take the residue of LSD out of the system, thereby helping eliminate recurrences.

Chaparral is high in protein, potassium, and sodium. It also contains silicon, tin, aluminum, sulphur, chlorine, and barium.

Aches

Acne

Allergies

ARTHRITIS

Backaches, chronic

BLOOD PURIFIER

Boils

Bowels, lower

Bruises
Bursitis
CANCER
Cataracts
Colds
Cuts
Eczema
Eyes (strengthens)
Hemorrhoids
Kidney infection

LEUKEMIA
Prostate
Psoriasis
Respiratory system
Rheumatism
Stomach disorders
TUMORS
Uterus, prolapsed
Venereal diseases
Wounds

CHICKWEED (chĭk'-wēd)
(Stellaria media)
Parts used: The Herb

Chickweed is valuable for treating blood toxicity, fevers, and inflammation. The mucilage elements are known for stomach ulcers and inflamed bowels. Chickweed will help dissolve the plaque out of the blood vessels and fatty substances in the system. Chickweed is mild and has been used as a food as well as medicine. It strengthens the stomach and bowels. It has antiseptic properties when exposed to the blood, and has been called an effective anti-cancer agent. It is used as a poultice for boils, burns, skin diseases, sore eyes and swollen testes.

Chickweed is rich in iron, copper and vitamin C. It contains lots of calcium and sodium and has a high content of the B-complex vitamin. It contains vitamin D, some manganese, phosphorus, and zinc.

APPETITE DEPRESSANT
Arteriosclerosis
Asthma
BLEEDING
Blood poisoning
BLOOD PURIFIER
Bronchitis
Bruises
Bursitis

Cancer preventive
Colitis
Constipation
CONVULSIONS
Cramps
Eye infections
Gas
Hemorrhoids
Lung congestion

Mucus
OBESITY
Pleurisy
SKIN RASHES
Testicles (swollen)

Tissues (inflamed)
ULCERS
Water retention
Wounds

CHICORY   (chik'-a-rē)
(Cichorium intybus)
Parts used: The Herb and Root

Chicory has many of the constituents of dandelion. It was well known in ancient Rome as a food and blood purifier. Chicory tea helps eliminate unwanted phlegm from the stomach. and is useful as a tea for upset stomach. It is useful in uric acid conditions of gout, rheumatics and joint stiffness. It has been used as a wash for boils and sores. It has been said that regular use of the tea is recommended for gallstones. The sap of the stems are used for poison ivy and sunburned skin.

It is rich in vitamins A, C, G, B, K, and P.

Anemia
Arteriosclerosis
Arthritis
BLOOD PURIFIER
CALCIUM DEPOSITS
Congestion
DIGESTION
Gallstones
Gout
Glands

Infertility
Inflammations
JAUNDICE
Kidney problems
LIVER PROBLEMS
PHLEGM (EXPELS)
Poultice
Rheumatism
Spleen problems
Tonic

CHINCHONA   (chin-chōn'-a)
(Cinchona calisaya)
Parts used: Bark

Chinchona contains quinine, which suppresses cell enzymes and acts as a disinfectant in cases of malaria and rheumatism. It is an effective preventative for influenza. It is one of the best tonics. It is used in all febrile and typhoid conditions and in remittent and intermittent fevers. It is very strengthening to the stomach in convalescence, and on the entire central nervous system. The liquid extract has been used as a cure for drunkeness.

Dropsy	Menstrual problems
FEVERS, INTERMITTENT	Measles
FLU	Nervous disorders
Heart palpitations	PARASITES
Hysteria	Rheumatism
Influenza preventative	Scrofula
MALARIA	Smallpox
JAUNDICE	Typhoid fever

CLOVES   (klōvz)
(Eugenia caryophyllata)
Parts used: Seeds

Cloves contain one of the most powerful germicidal agents in the herb kingdom. It is safe and effective for vomiting during pregnancy, and increases circulation of the blood and promotes digestion and nutrition. The oil of cloves is a diffusive stimulant and is often rubbed on the gums to relieve toothache and is frequently used as a remedy for bad breath.

Cloves contain vitamins C and A, the B-complex vitamin and contain potassium, phosphorus, calcium, magnesium and sodium.

BAD BREATH	GAS
Blood pressure, low	Indigestion
BRONCHIAL CATARRH	NAUSEA
CIRCULATION, POOR	Pain
Colitis (mucus)	Palsy
Diarrhea	Spasms
DIZZINESS	Toothache
Dysentery	VOMITING
EARACHE	Sexual stimulant
Epilepsy	

COLTSFOOT (kŏlts'-füt)
(Tussilago farfara)
Parts used: Leaves

Coltsfoot is known as a remedy for coughs and respiratory ailments. The ingredients of the flowers are chiefly expectorant in effect, being very soothing to the mucous membranes. It has a soothing effect on the throat as well as on the brains' cough-activating mechanism. It is a chest and lung expectorant. Coltsfoot contains a high percentage of mucilage and saponins which have disinfectant and anti-inflammatory effects on respiratory problems. Used with horehound and marshmallow Coltsfoot is one of the best cough remedies. Use as a tea.

It is rich in vitamins A and C, but also contains calcium, potassium, vitamin P, zinc, B_{12}, and B_6. There are traces of manganese, iron and copper in Coltsfoot.

ASTHMA
BRONCHITIS
CATARRAH
Chills
Colds
COUGHS
Diarrhea
Emphysema
Hoarseness

Inflammation
LUNG PROBLEMS
MUCUS
Pleurisy
Pneumonia
Swellings
Tracheitis (calms)
Tuberculosis
WHOOPING COUGHS

COMFREY (kŭm'-frē)
(Symphytum officinale)
Parts used: Leaves and Roots

Comfrey is one of the most valuable herbs known to botanic medicine. It has been used for centuries with success as a wound-healer and bone knitter. It feeds the pituitary with its natural hormone and helps strengthen the body skeleton. It helps in the calcium-phosphorus balance by promoting strong bones and healthy skin. It helps promote the secretion of pepsin and is a general aid to digestion. It has a beneficial effect on all parts of the body, being used as an over all tonic. It is one of the finest healers for the respiratory system, and can be used both internally and externally for healing of fractures, wounds, sores and ulcers. It has been used with great success to check hemorrhage, whether from the stomach, lungs, bowels, kidneys or piles.

Comfrey is rich in vitamins A and C. It is high in calcium, potassium, phosphorus, and protein. It contains iron, magnesium, sulphur, copper and zinc, as well as eighteen Amino acids. It is a good source of the amino acid, hysine, usually lacking in diets that contain no animal products.

Allergies	Fatigue
ANEMIA	FRACTURES
ARTHRITIS	Gangrene
Asthma	Gout
Bladder	Hay fever
Bleeding	Infections
BLOOD CLEANSER	Insect bites
BOILS	Kidney stones
BREAKS	Leg cramps
Bronchitis	LUNGS
BRUISES	Pain
BURNS	Pleurisy
Bursitis	Pneumonia
Cancer	Respiratory problems
Colds	Sinusitis
Colitis	Skin trouble
Coughs	SORES
Cramps	SPRAINS
Diarrhea	Stomach trouble
Digestion	SWELLING
EMPHYSEMA	Tonic
Eczema	Tuberculosis

CORNSILK (kôrn-sĭlk)
(Stigmata maidis)
Parts used: Silk

Cornsilk is used for complaints of the bladder. Physicians have used it as a diuretic and conditions of cystitis. It has a cleansing effect on the circulation of urea and is valuable in the treatment of renal and cystic inflammations. It will cleanse the cystic membrane in cystic catarrh and will manifest antiseptic powers in morbid deposits.

Cornsilk is rich in vitamin K. It also contains vitamin B, PABA, and silicon.

Arteriosclerosis	HEART TROUBLE
Bedwetting	High blood pressure
BLADDER PROBLEMS	KIDNEY PROBLEMS
Cholesterol	Obesity
Cystic irritation	Prostate
Gonorrhea	Urinary problems

COUCH GRASS (kouch grās)
(Agropyron repens)
Parts used: The Herb

Couch Grass is well known for its beneficial effects on the urinary system. It is a good spring tonic. It is used for early stages of catarrhal troubles. Couch Grass is especially used in cystitis and the treatment of catarrhal diseases of the bladder. It has been known to help eliminate stones and gravel from the kidneys and bladder. The extracts are known to have antibiotic effects against a variety of bacteria and molds.

Couch Grass is rich in vitamins A, C, and the B-complex vitamins. It is high in silicon, potassium, and sodium, and contains smaller amounts of magnesium and calcium.

BLADDER INFECTIONS
BLOOD PURIFIER
Bright's disease
Bronchitis
CATARRHAL
    CONDITIONS
Constipation
CYSTITIS
Eyes (strengthens)
Female disorders
Fevers
Gout

Gravel
JAUNDICE
KIDNEY PROBLEMS
Lumbago
Lungs
Prostate glands
RHEUMATISM
Skin diseases
Syphilis
TONIC
URINARY INFECTIONS

CRAMP BARK   (krămp bärk)
(Viburnum opulus)
Parts used: Bark and Berries

Cramp Bark is considered one of the best female regulators in nature. It has been recommended to help prevent nervous diseases of pregnancy, after-pains, and cramps, especially the nervous discomforts of pregnancy. Cramp Bark is considered a very valuable herb. It is recognized as a uterine sedative and anti-spasmodic. It is the best relaxant to the ovaries and uterus. In Russia, the berries are used fresh or dried for high blood pressure, heart problems (with seeds), coughs, colds, lungs, kidneys, and bleeding and stomach ulcers. Externally, a decoction of flowers have been used for eczema and other skin conditions.

It contains potassium, calcium and magnesium. The berry is sometimes used like cranberries. They are very rich in vitamins C and K, along with some minerals.

ASTHMA
Colic
Constipation
CONVULSIONS
CRAMPS
Dysentery

Epilepsy
Fainting
Fits
Gallstones
Gas
HEART PALPITATION

HYPERTENSION	Neuralgia
HYSTERIA	Ovarian irritations
Jaundice	Pregnancy (after pains)
LEG CRAMPS	Pulse (regulates)
Lock jaw	Rheumatism
Miscarriage	SPASMS
NERVOUSNESS	URINARY PROBLEMS

CULVER'S ROOT (kul'-verz rüt)
(Varoniscastrum virgincum)
Parts used: Root

Culver's Root has a gentle relaxant and tonic effect on the liver. It is considered a tonic for the stomach. It also helps intestinal indigestion, purifies the blood, and removes morbid catarrhal obstructions and congestions in a mild, natural way. Culver's Root should be taken with an herb that helps expel gas such as fennel. Its action is similar to Mandrake but concentrates on the duodenum. Mandrake acts more on the liver, stimulating it to produce more bile.

Culver's Root contains potassium and magnesium.

BLOOD PURIFIER	Food poisoning
CATARRHAL	LIVER PROBLEMS
OBSTRUCTIONS	Scrofulous diseases
DIARRHEA	STOMACH PROBLEMS
Fevers	Syphlitic diseases

CYANI or CORNFLOWER (sī'-ăn-ē)
(Centaurea cyanus)
Parts used: The Herb

Cornflower was used by the Plains Indians as an antidote for snakebites, insect bites and stings. The properties have action similar to that of Blessed Thistle. Its nervine powers are highly rated by herbalists. The water distilled from cornflower petals has been used as a remedy for weak eyes. The dried powder can be used on bruises. The seeds, leaves or the distilled water of the herb taken in wine is very good against the plague and all infectious diseases. It is good for ulcers and sores in the mouth. Cornflower is used as a remedy in certain forms of temporary paralysis.

CONJUNCTIVITIS   Infection
CORNEAL ULCERS   Mumps
Dermatitis   NERVOUS DISORDERS
DISEASES   POISONOUS BITES
EYE DISORDERS   Sight (weak)
Fevers, pestilential   STINGS
Indigestion, chronic   Toothache

DAMIANA   (dăm-i-ă'-nă)
(Turnera aphrodisiaca)
Parts used: Leaves

Damiana has stimulating properties and has been used for nervousness, weakness and exhaustion. Damiana has been recommended for increasing sperm count in the male, and to strengthen the egg in the female. It helps to balance the hormones in women. In Mexico, it is used for female disorders. It is especially beneficial for an exhausted state of the body and of the vital powers of the system. It is useful in increasing sexual prowess in persons who suffer from sexual weakness.

It has been used as a mild tonic laxative for children.

Damiana has been said to be one of the most popular and safest of all plants claimed to restore the natural sexual capacities and functions.

Brain tonic
BRONCHITIS
Energy
EMPHYSEMA
Exhaustion
Female problems
Frigidity

HORMONE BALANCER
HOT FLASHES
MENOPAUSE
Nervousness
PARKINSON'S DISEASE
Prostate
SEXUAL STIMULANT

DANDELION   (dan'-da-līán)
(Taraxacum officinale)
Parts used: Leaves and Roots

Dandelion benefits the function of the liver. It has the ability to clear obstructions and stimulates the liver to detoxify poisons. It should be considered a valuable survival food. It contains all the nutritive salts that are required for the body to purify the blood. It promotes a healthy circulation, strengthens weak arteries, cleanses skin blemishes and restores the gastric balance in patients who have suffered from severe vomiting.

The juice of the broken stem can be applied to warts and allowed to dry. If used daily for two or three days, it will dry up the warts. It is also useful for corns, acne and blisters.

A diet of this herb (green) improves the enamel of the teeth.

Dandelion is a natural source of protein. It is rich in vitamin A. It is an excellent source of vitamin B., C and E. It is rich in potassium, calcium and sodium. It contains some phosphorus and iron, as well as some nickel, cobalt, tin, copper, and zinc.

Age spots
ANEMIA
BLISTERS, EXTERNAL
BLOOD PRESSURE
  (LOWERS)
BLOOD PURIFIER
Constipation

Corns
Cramps
Dermatitis
Diabetes
Eczema
ENDURANCE
Fatigue

Fever
GALL BLADDER
Gout
Jaundice
Hypoglycemia
LIVER PROBLEMS

Metabolism (stimulates)
Psoriasis
Rheumatism
Spleen
Stomach
Warts

DEVILS CLAW   (dev'als klō)
(Harpagophytum procumbens)
Parts used: Root

Devils Claw has been proven with extensive experiments to have healing powers in arthritis, rheumatism, diabetes, arteriosclerosis, and liver, kidney and bladder diseases. It has properties similar to chaparral, which has the ability to cleanse deep into the muscles and tissue walls. It has natural cleansing agents to clean the system of toxic impurities.

Experiments have shown that regular use of the decoction will help the hardened vascular walls once again to become elastic, and there is a generalized feeling of strength, which seem to improve the complaints of old age.

One doctor suggests using Devils Claw once a year for the healthy person, especially during the spring, to cleanse the most important organs, lymph and blood.

ARTERIOSCLEROSIS
ARTHRITIS
BLADDER
 (STRENGTHENS)
BLOOD PURIFIER
CHOLESTEROL
DIABETES
Gallstones

Gout
KIDNEYS
 (STRENGTHENS)
LIVER DISEASES
Malaria
POLLUTION (AIR)
RHEUMATISM
STOMACH PROBLEMS

DONG QUAI   (dön kwī′)
(Angelica sinensis)
Parts used: Root

Dong Quai has been named the queen of all female herbs. This herb has a tranquilizing effect on the central nervous system and gives nourishment to the brain cells. It nourishes the blood, lubricates the intestines, and promotes the growth of the womb. Dong Quai has been acclaimed to be very effective against almost every type of complaint of the female system. It possesses constituents for nourishing female glands, and helps to strengthen all internal body organs and muscles. It also helps to rebuild the blood and improve the conditions of the mother-to-be.

It helps to dissolve blood clots and to loosen tight muscles. It is a good blood purifier and cleanser, helping to increase circulation. It is useful in aiding recovery from an accident if internal bleeding and body bruises exist.

This herb contains vitamin A, B12, and E.

Abdominal ache	Headaches, migraine
Aches	HOT FLASHES
ANEMIA	Hypertension
Angina	Hypoglycemia
BLEEDING, INTERNAL	Lumbago
BLOOD PURIFIER	MENOPAUSE
BRAIN NOURISHER	MENSTRUATION (REG-
Bruises	ULATOR)
Chills	Metabolism
Circulation	NERVOUSNESS
Clots (blood)	Preventive
Constipation	Stomach
Cramps	Tonic
FEMALE GLANDS	Tumors (blood)

ECHINACEA   (i-kī-nā'-sē-a)
(Echinacea augustifolia)
Parts used: Root

Echinacea stimulates the immune response, increasing the body's ability to resist infections, especially the production of white blood cells. It improves lymphatic filtration and drainage, and it helps remove toxins from the blood. It is considered one of the best blood cleansers and is called the King of the Blood Purifiers. It is considered a non-toxic way of cleansing the system. It is said to be good for enlargement and weakness of the prostate gland. It is a natural antibiotic. It has been used with Chickweed to help in weight loss.

It contains vitamins A, E, and C, iron, iodine, copper, sulphur, and potassium.

Acne	Gums
Antiseptic	Hydrophobia
Bites, poisonous	Indigestion
BLOOD BUILDER	INFECTIONS, EXTERNAL
BLOOD DISEASES	INFECTIONS (PREVENTS)
BLOOD POISONING	Leukemia
BLOOD PURIFIER	LYMPH GLANDS
BOILS	Mucus
Cancer	Peritonitis
Carbuncle	Pimples
Diphtheria	PROSTATE
Eczema	Sores, infected
Fevers	Strep throat
Gangrene	Syphilis
Glands, swollen	Typhoid fever
Gonorrhea	Tonsillitis

ELDER FLOWER (el' dĕr flow' ĕr)
(Sambucus nigra)
Parts used: Flowers and Berries

Elder Flower is considered one of the greatest and most versatile herbs in the treatment of disease. Its result is seen in the ability of the herb to detoxify the body cells of toxic waste. It increases blood circulation and promotes sweating. It will bring down fever when needed.

It is an alterative, blood purifier and cell cleanser. Elder Flower contains constituents that act as sedatives and relieve pain. It works as an expectorant and an anti-catarrhal action and anti-inflammatory agent. It is a wonderful remedy for babies, children, adults and the elderly.

Elder Flower and peppermint blend well together to combat colds, flu and fevers. For infections, it is excellent when combined with golden seal and yarrow. For lung congestion or asthma it works well when combined with mullein. For an eyewash Elder Flower blends well with eyebright and golden seal.

Elder Flower contains vitamin A, C and bioflavonoids.

ALLERGIES	Flu
ASTHMA	Gas
Brain inflammation	HAY FEVER
BRONCHITIS	Hemorrhoids
Cancer	Joints, swollen
COLDS	Nerves
Digestive problems	PNEUMONIA
Ear infections	SINUS CONGESTION
Eye infections	Skin diseases
Eye strain	Ulcers
FEVERS	

ELECAMPANE   (el-i-kam-pān')
(Inula helenium)
Parts used: Root

Elecampane has been used for intestinal worms, retention of water, and to lessen tooth decay and firm the gums. It is also used for any catarrh conditions. It gives relief to respiratory difficulties and assists expectoration and general catarrhal conditions. Elecampane is one of the richest sources of natural insulin, and is therefore helpful for the pancreas. It is usually preferred in combination with other herbs. It has antiseptic properties and is used in Spain as a surgical dressing and as an antiseptic in surgery.
It contains calcium, potassium and sodium.

Asthma	Disposition (helper)
Assimilation, poor	Female problems
Bladder catarrh	Lungs
BRONCHITIS, CHRONIC	Menstrual problems
Colic	Phlegm (expels)
Consumption	Poison, counteracts
Convulsions	Stomach tonic
COUGHS	Urethra (catarrhal)
Cramps	Whooping cough
Digestion	Worms

EPHEDRA (Brigham Tea)   (i-fed'-ra)
(Ephedra species)
Parts used: The Herb

Ephedra (Brigham Tea) is closely related to adrenaline and has some of the same properties. It stimulates the nervous system and acts directly on the muscle cells. It is used in the Soviet Union for treating rheumatism and syphilis. The juice of the berry has been given for respiratory problems. Ephedra

contains substances that effect the blood vessels, all the small
blood vessels, especially the small arteries and capillaries. Its
effect on the heart causes slower and stronger beat. It is considered a bronchial dilator and decongestant.

It contains some vitamin B12, cobalt, strontium, nickel,
and copper.

Arthritis	HEADACHES
Asthma	Heart palpitations
Bleeding, internal	Joint problems
Blood pressure (normalizes)	KIDNEYS
BLOOD PURIFIER	Menstruation
BRONCHITIS	Muscle problems
BURSITIS	Nosebleeds
Colds	Pain
Depression	Pneumonia
Diphtheria	Scarlet fever
Drug overdose	Sinus
Fever	Skin diseases
Gall bladder	Tonic
Hayfever	VENEREAL DISEASE

EUCALYPTUS (yoo'-ka-lip'-tas)
(Eucalyptus globulus)
Parts used: Oil

Eucalyptus has antiseptic properties in the leaves. It is very
potent but safe to use. The oil is useful with pyorrhea and burns
to prevent infections. It is helpful against poisonous germs.
Eucalyptus trees have been planted in fever districts and marshy
areas infected with mosquitoes, and found that its leaves con-
vert the oxygen of the air into ozone. It is also found to be a great
life-giver, purifier, vitalizer, and sweetener of all organic matter.

The oil can be snuffed to clear sinus congestion. Oil mixed
with water is good for insect repellant. Small drop on the tongue
will help nausea.

Asthma	Nausea
Boils, external	NEURALGIA
BRONCHITIS	Paralysis
Burns (oil)	Piles
Cancer	PYORRHEA (OIL)
Carbuncles, external	SORES, EXTERNAL
Catarrh	Throat, sore
Croup	Typhoid
Diptheria	Ulcers, external
Fever	Uterus, prolapsed
Indigestion	Worms
LUNGS	WOUNDS
Malarial diseases	

EVENING PRIMROSE   (ēv'-ning prim'-rōz)
(Oenothera biennis)
Parts used: Bark, Leaves Oil

Evening Primrose stimulates the action of the stomach to help in liver and spleen conditions. It works on alimentary toxins due to a faulty diet which may affect the central nervous system. It has been used in Europe to treat Multiple Sclerosis. It contains hormone-like substances called prostaglandins called miracle molecules. It stops thrombosis and lowers blood pressure. It also opens up blood vessels and relieves the pain of angina. It slows down the speed at which cholesterol is made and has been found to be effective in lowering cholesterol levels, in inhibiting the formation of clots and in lowering blood pressure in those with mild to moderate hypertension. It prevents inflammation and controls arthritis. In the laboratory, Evening Primrose stops the growth of numerous kinds of cancer cells.

Evening Primrose contains minerals and is high in potassium and magnesium.

Alcoholism	Asthma, spasmodic
Allergies	Bowel problems
Arthritis	Cancer

Colds
COUGHS, NERVOUS
Cramps, menstrual
Female disorders
Glaucoma
Headaches, migraine
HIGH BLOOD PRESSURE
Hyperactivity (in children)
Mental depression

Multiple sclerosis
NERVES
Neuralgia
Obesity
Sedative effect
Skin irritation
Ulcers
WHOOPING COUGH

EYEBRIGHT (ī'-brīt')
(Euphrasia officinalis)
Parts used: The Herb

Eyebright aids in stimulating the liver to clean the blood and relieve the conditions that effect the clarity of vision and thought. It is useful for inflammations because of its cooling and detoxifying properties. It has antiseptic properties that fight infections of the eyes. It has traditionally been used as a remedy for eye problems, such as failing vision, eye inflammation, conjunctivitis, ulcers and even eye strain. Eyebright will strengthen all parts of the eye and provide an elasticity to the nerves and optic devices responsible for sight.

It is extremely rich in vitamins A and C. It contains B complex, vitamin D, and some vitamin E. It also contains iron, silicon, a trace of iodine, copper, and zinc.

Black eye compress
BLOOD CLEANSER
CATARACTS
Catarrh
COLDS
Congestion
Coughs
Earache
Eye disorders and infections
Eye problems

EYE (STRENGTHENS)
Hay fever
Headaches and colds
Head colds
Hoarseness
LIVER STIMULANT
Memory
Sinus congestion
Styes (dissolves)

FALSE UNICORN   (fôls yōō'-na-kôrn')
(Chamaelirium luteum)
Parts used: Root

False Unicorn is an excellent overall tonic. It is useful to the mucous membranes and a delicate stomach. It has been said that it is as good as pumpkin seeds for the removal of tapeworms. It contains strong turpentine constituents and antiseptic principles. False Unicorn stimulates reproductive organs in men and women. It has been used to correct almost all problems of the reproductive organs of male and female. This herb is important for menopausal problems because of its effect in uterine disorders, headaches and depression.

False Unicorn is high in vitamin C. It also contains copper, sulphur, cadmium, cobalt, molybdenum, and traces of zinc.

Appetite stimulant	Headaches
Bright's disease	KIDNEYS
COLIC	Menopause
COUGHS	MISCARRIAGE
Depression	(PREVENTS)
Diabetes	Nausea
DIGESTIVE PROBLEMS	Ovaries
Dropsy	PROSTATE
Dyspepsia	Side pain
Enuresis	TAPEWORM
Gastro-intestinal weaknesses	Uterine problems

FENNEL   (fĕn'-al)
(Foeniculum valgare)
Parts used: Seeds

Fennel helps to take away the appetite. When boiled with barley, it aids lactation. It helps stabilize the nervous system and moves waste material out of the body. It has an anticonvulsive and pain-relieving property and is recommended as a sedative for small children. Fennel improves digestion and has a diuretic effect. It is also helpful in cases of cough and persistent bronchitis, with its mucus-countering and anticonvulsive properties. Fennel contains potassium, sulphur and sodium.

Appetite depressant	GAS
Bronchitis	Gout
COLIC	INTESTINAL PROBLEMS
Congestion	Lactation (promotes)
Convulsions	Nervous disorders
Coughs	Pin worms
Cramps, abdominal	SEDATIVE FOR CHIL-
Digestive aid	DREN
Female problems	Spasms

FENUGREEK (fĕn-yōō-grēk')
(Trigonella foenum-graecum)
Parts used: Seeds

Fenugreek has the ability to soften and dissolve hardened masses of accumulated mucus. It helps to expel toxic waste through the lymphatic system. It expels mucus and phlegm from the bronchial tubes. It has antiseptic properties and kills infections in the lungs. Fenugreek contains lecithin which dissolves cholesterol and contains lipotropic (fat dissolving) substances, which dissolve deposits of fat, prevents fatty accumulations, and water retention. The constituents in the seeds contain a saponin closely related to those in yucca. Fenugreek used with lemon juice and honey soothes and nourishes the body and helps to reduce fevers.

It is rich in vitamins A and D. It also contains an oil that resembles cod liver oil. Fenugreek is rich in minerals and is high in protein also. It has vitamins B_1, B_2 and B_3 and contains choline, lecithin, and iron.

Abscess	Blood poisoning
Bad breath	Boils

Body odor   LUNG INFECTIONS
BRONCHIAL CATARRH   MUCUS (DISSOLVES)
Carbuncles   STOMACH IRRITATIONS
CHOLESTEROL   Throat gargle
   (DISSOLVES)   Ulcers
Fevers (reduce)   Uterus
Inflammations   Water retention
Lactation   Wounds (poultice)

FEVERFEW   (fĕ' vēr-few)
(Chrysanthemum parthenium)
Parts used: Leaves and flowers.

Feverfew is not a new herb, it is a rediscovered one, being a natural remedy for pain relief. It is considered the best remedy for the worst headaches. It was used in the past as aspirin and codeine are used today. It was used in ague (a fever of malarial origin), or any ailment where chills, fever or headaches developed.

Feverfew is a natural relief for migraine headaches. It is excellent for relieving colds, and in inflammation from arthritis. It is used in dizziness, tinnitus and aids in circulation to the brain and head area.

Feverfew contains elements that work synergistically to regulate normal function of the body. It works gradually and with gentler action allowing the body to heal itself. It works in a natural way to strengthen the body.

Feverfew contains high amounts of iron, niacin, manganese, phosphorus, potassium, and selenium. It also contains vitamin A, C, silicon, sodium and zinc.

Aches   Arthritis
Ague   CHILLS
Allergies   Circulation

COLDS
Digestion
Dizziness
Female problems
HEADACHES
Hot flashes
Insect bites (external)
Menopause symptoms

Menstruation (promotes)
MIGRAINE HEADACHES
Nervous headaches
Nervous hysteria
PAIN
SINUS HEADACHES
Tinnitus
Vertigo

FIGWORT   (fig'-wòrt)
(Scrophularia nodosa)
Parts used: The Herb and Root

Figwort provides hormone-like materials into the system to help soothe the digestive organs. This also cleans the kidneys. Figwort has an effect on the entire body. It is used as a poultice for ulcers, piles, scrofulous glands in the neck, sores and wounds and toothache. In Wales, it is used to treat circulatory disorders and is especially good at reducing varicose veins. It is said Figwort will lessen high blood pressure, and is a diuretic as well as an efficient pain killer when nothing stronger is at hand. It is essentially a skin medication used for eczema, scabies, tumors and rashes.

ABRASIONS
Anxiety
ATHLETE'S FOOT
Burns
CRADLE CAP
Cuts
Digestive organs
Eczema
FEVER
Hemorrhoids

IMPETIGO
Insomnia
Kidneys
Menstrual flow (increases)
Nightmares
RESTLESSNESS
SKIN DISEASES
TUMORS (SKIN)
Worms

FLAXSEED   (flăks'-sēd')
(Linum usitatissimum)
Parts used: Seeds

Flaxseed is a natural laxative. It is soothing and provides roughage with mucilaginous qualities. It heals the body as it nourishes and is soothing to the throat, entire stomach and intestinal linings. It has been used for weakly babies, enriching the blood, and strengthening the nerves. It is used as a poultice and compresses with herbal medication, applied as hot as one can stand it.

Flaxseed contains calcium and potassium.

Bronchitis	Liver complaint
CATARRH (CONDITIONS)	Lung problems
Colds	Pleurisy
CONSTIPATION	Pneumonia
Gallstones	Rheumatism, muscular
Heart (strengthens)	Worms
Jaundice	

GARLIC   (gär-lĭk)
(Allium sativum)
Parts used: Bulb

Garlic is nature's antibiotic. The properties of garlic have the ability of stimulating cell growth and activity. It has a rejuvenative effect on all body functions. It is a health building and disease preventative herb and dissolves cholesterol in the bloodstream. Garlic stimulates the lymphatic system to throw off waste materials. Garlic opens up the blood vessels and reduces blood pressure in hypertensive patients. It contains antibiotics that are effective against bacteria which may be resistant to other antibiotics. It is called Russian penicillin. Garlic does not destroy the body's normal flora.

This herb contains vitamins A and C. It also contains selenium, which is closely related to vitamin E in biological activity. It contains sulphur, calcium, manganese, copper, and a lot of vitamin B₁. Garlic also contains some iron and it is high in potassium and zinc.

Anemia	Hypoglycemia
Arthritis	Infections
Allergies	INFECTIOUS DISEASE
ASTHMA	INTESTINAL WORMS
CANCER IMMUNITY	Insomnia
Catarrh	Memory
Cold congestion	Mucus
Diabetes	Parasites
DIGESTIVE DISORDERS	Regulator of glands
EAR INFECTIONS	Skin problems
Emphysema	Toothache
Fevers	Toxic metal poisoning
Germ killer	Warts
Heart disease	Worms
HIGH BLOOD PRESSURE	Yeast infection
Hypertension	

GENTIAN (jĕn-shăn)
(Gentiana lutea)
Parts used: Root

Gentian is superior to other herbal aids because it does not cause constipation. It stimulates the circulation and strengthens the system, being one of the best stomach tonics in the herb kingdom. Gentian is rich in natural sugar and is useful for strengthening the pancreas and the spleen, as well as the kidneys. It is used for weakened muscular tone of the digestive organs, and as an appetite stimulant and is helpful for convalescing and weak patients.

Gentian is high in iron. It contains B-complex especially inositol and niacin. It contains Vitamin F, manganese, silicon, sulphur, tin, lead, and zinc.

Amenorrhea	Heartburn
Anemia	HYSTERIA
Antidote for poisons	JAUNDICE
APPETITE STIMULANT	Joint inflammation
Bites (mad dog)	LIVER BILE
Blood (strengthens)	Nausea
Bruises	Scrofula
Constipation	Spleen disorders
Cramps	Stomach problems
Debility	Sprains
Diarrhea	Urinary infection
Female weakness	Vermin
Fevers	Worms
Gout	Wounds (infected)

GINGER   (jǐn'-jar)
(Zingiber officinale)
Parts used: Root

Ginger is an excellent herb for the respiratory system. It is good for fighting off colds and flu. It removes congestion, relieves headaches and aches and pains, and helps to clear sore throats. It is excellent for upset stomach and indigestion. It is very effective as a cleansing agent through the bowels and kidneys and also through the skin. Ginger is an excellent herb to combine with other herbs to enhance their effectiveness. It can also be added to meat dishes to help the intestines to detoxify the meat. Ginger and capsium work together for bronchial congestion and stuffy noses.

It contains protein, vitamins A, C and B-complex. It also contains calcium, phosphorus, iron, sodium, potassium and magnesium.

Bowels (spasms)
Bronchitis
CHILDHOOD DISEASES
CIRCULATION
COLDS
COLIC
Colitis
Coughs
Diarrhea
Dropsy
Female obstruction
FEVERS
FLU
GAS PAINS

HEADACHE
Heart palpitations
INDIGESTION
Lung problems
Menstruation (promotes)
MORNING SICKNESS
Nausea
Nervous problems
Perspiration (promotes)
STOMACH (SETTLES)
Throat, sore
TONIC
TOOTHACHE
WHOOPING COUGH

GINKGO (gink' gō)
(Ginkgo biloba)
Parts used:

European studies have shown that Ginkgo increases blood flow in the brain to improve memory and help prevent and treat strokes by preventing formation of blood clots. French scientists found positive results when using Ginkgo for natural blood clotting, arterial blood flow, asthma attacks and even organ transplant rejection.

This herb helps arteries in the legs and relieves pain, cramping and weakness, It increases circulation of blood flow in the retina and prevents muscular degeneration. Ear problems are improved with Ginkgo, due to improved blood flow to the nerves of the inner ear. It is found to benefit chronic ringing in the ears (tinnitus).

Ginkgo is a gift for the aging. It increases oxygen and blood flow to the brain and extremities, improves mental clarity and inhibits free radical scavengers from destroying cells. It supplies nutritional support to all areas of the body. It dilates the blood vessels, allowing improved blood flow to the tissues. It eliminates waste material and inhibits the clumping of blood platelets, and prevents circulating platelets from sticking together, which contributes to heart problems, strokes and artery conditions.

Ginkgo is an adaptogen herb, which helps the body deal with stressful situations.

Allergies	Heart problems
ALZHEIMER'S	Lung problems
Alertness	MEMORY LOSS
Anxiety attacks	Mental clarity
Arthritis	Mood swings
Asthma	Muscular degenestration
ATTENTION SPAN	Raynauds' Disease
CIRCULATORY DISORDERS	STROKE
Cancer	Tinnitus
Coughs	Toxic Shock Syndrome
Depression	Varicose veins
DIZZINESS	Vascular impotence
Equilibrium problems	Vertigo
Headaches	

GINSENG (jĭn'-sĕng')
Korean (Panax schin-seng) Siberian (Eleutherococcus) Wild American (panax quinquefolium)
Parts used: Root

In the Orient Ginseng is called the King of the Herbs. It stimulates the entire body energy to overcome stress, fatigue, and weakness. It is especially stimulating for mental fatigue. It stimulates and improves the brain cells. Ginseng has a very beneficial effect on the heart and circulation. It is used to normalize blood pressure, reduce blood cholesterol and prevent arteriosclerosis. It is used as a preventive tonic in China. It is claimed to slow down the aging process. It is considered a cure-all herb. It acts as an antidote to various types of drugs and toxic chemicals, and is said to protect the body against radiation. It is said to improve vision and hearing activity, improve working ability, and help to check irritability to give one more poise and composure.

Ginseng contains vitamins A and E. It also contains thiamine, riboflavin, B_{12}, niacin, calcium, iron, phosphorus, sodium, silicon, potassium, manganese, magnesium, sulphur, and tin.

AGE SPOTS
Anemia
Antidote for some drugs
Appetite
Bleeding, internal
Blood diseases
BLOOD PRESSURE
Childbirth (bleeding)
DEPRESSION
Digestive problems
ENDURANCE
 (INCREASES)
Euphoria (induces)
Fatigue (banishes)
Fevers
HEMORRHAGE
Inflammation
Irritability (helps)
Liver diseases
LONGEVITY
Lung problems
Menopause
Menstruation
Mental vigor

Nausea   SEXUAL STIMULANT
Nervousness   STRESS
PHYSICAL VIGOR   Ulcers
Radiation protection   Vomiting

GLUCOMANNAN   (glŭ-cō-măn-nun)
(Amorphophallus konjak)
Part used: Root

Glucomannan is high in fiber, essential for cleaning the digestive system. Glucomannan is taken from the Konjac root and is from the same family as the yam, which is 100 percent natural dietary fiber without calories. Since lack of fiber is a major cause for the high incidence of growing gastrointestinal disorders, it is a valuable herb.

It helps reduce cholesterol, helps maintain regularity and promotes bowel health. It helps to normalize blood sugar, to relieve stress on the pancreas and to discourage blood sugar abnormalities, such as hypoglycemia.

Glucomannan absorbs toxic substances produced during digestion and elimination. It binds toxic material and eliminates them before they can be absorbed into the blood stream.

Glucomannan and lecithin together are food supplements found in clinical studies to be useful in reducing cholesterol levels. Lecithin regulates metabolism and breaks down fat and cholesterol preventing adhering to the artery walls, while Glucomannan eliminates it out of the body.

This herb acts as a prevention of chronic disease and a weight control agent. As a diet aid, it expands to about 50 times its original volume when used with a large glass of water.

Glucomannan contains Vitamins A, C, niacin, B1 and B2. It also contains calcium, magnesium, phosphorus, potassium, sodium, iron, zinc, selenium, manganese and silicon.

Atherosclerosis	HEMORRHOIDS
CONSTIPATION	High blood pressure
Diabetes	Hypoglycemia
Digestive problems	OBESITY
DIVERTICULAR DISEASE	Pancreas (reduces stress)

GOLDEN SEAL (gōl'-den sēl')
(Hydrastis canadensis)
Parts used: Rhizome and Root

Golden Seal has been recommended as a way of boosting a sluggish glandular system and promoting youthful hormone harmony. The action of the herb goes directly into the bloodstream and helps regulate the liver functions. It has a natural antibiotic ability to stop infection and kill poisons in the body. It should not be used by pregnant women. Golden Seal can be used for many illnesses not listed.

Golden Seal is valuable for all catarrhal conditions either in the nasal area, bronchial tubes, throat, intestines, stomach and bladder. It has the ability to heal mucous membranes anywhere in the body. It ranks high as one of the best general medicinal aids in the herbal kingdom. When taken with other herbs, it increases the tonic properties for whatever ailment is being treated. If a person has low blood sugar, substitute **myrrh** instead of Golden Seal.

This herb contains vitamins A and C. It also contains vitamin B-complex, E, F, calcium, copper, potassium, lots of phosphorus, manganese, iron, zinc and sodium.

ANTIBIOTIC	INFECTION
ANTISEPTIC	Insect repellent
BLEEDING, INTERNAL	LIVER PROBLEMS
Cancer	MENSTRUATION,
Catarrh	EXCESSIVE
COLON INFLAMMATION	Morning sickness
Constipation, chronic	MOUTH SORES
Eczema	Ringworm
EYE INFECTIONS	Rhinitis
Gastritis	Skin problems
Genital disorders	Tonsillitis
Gonorrhea	Ulceration, skin
HEMORRHAGING,	Urethritis
INTERNAL	VAGINITIS
Herpes simplex, genital	Venereal disease

GOTU KOLA   (gȯt-ū kō'-lā)
(Hydrocotyle asiatica)
Parts used: The Herb

Gotu Kola is good when used after a nervous breakdown. It is able to rebuild energy reserves. For this reason, it is called 'food for the brain'. It increases mental and physical power. It combats stress and improves reflexes. Gotu Kola has an energizing effect on the cells of the brain. It is said also to help prevent nervous breakdown. It relieves high blood pressure, mental fatigue, and senility, and helps the body defend itself against various toxins.

Gotu Kola contains vitamins A, G, and K and is high in magnesium. It probably contains vitamins E and some B and minerals, but at this point no research has been done in the United States.

Blood purifier
Bowel problems
Depression
FATIGUE
Fevers
Heart (strengthens)
HIGH BLOOD PRESSURE
Infections
Leprosy
Longevity
Memory
Menopause

MENTAL FATIGUE
NERVOUS BREAKDOWN
PHYSICAL FATIGUE
Rheumatism
Scrofula
SENILITY
Thyroid stimulant
TONIC
Toxins (defense)
Vitality
Wounds

GUM WEED (gŭm wēd)
(Grindelia squarrosa)
Parts used: Flowering Top and Leaves

Gum Weed acts as an antidote for the treatment of poison oak and ivy. It can be used for all skin disorders. It has been used for the spasms of asthma and whooping cough for broncial irritations and nasal congestion. This should not be used when the heart is weak.

Gum Weed is high in selenium. It also contains lead, traces of arsenic, tin, cadmium and zinc.

ASTHMA
BRONCHITIS
BLADDER INFECTION
Blisters, external
Burns, external
Dermatitis, allergic
Eczema
Emphysema

Flu
Impetigo
POISON IVY AND OAK
PSORIASIS
SKIN DISORDERS
UTERUS INFECTION
WHOOPING COUGH

HAWTHORN (hô'-thôrn')
(Crategnus oxyacantha)
Parts used: Berries

Hawthorn is very effective for relieving insomnia. A poultice of leaves (crushed) or fruit has strong drawing powers and has been used in England for centuries in the treatment of embedded thorns, splinters, felons and whitlows. The fruits are used for nervousness and also in preventing miscarriage. It has been known for centuries as a treatment of heart disease. Regular use strengthens the heart muscles. It has been used in preventing arteriosclerosis and in helping conditions like rapid and feeble heart action, heart valve defects, enlarged heart, angina pectoris and difficult breathing owing to ineffective heart action and lack of oxygen in the blood. Some herbalists recommend Hawthorn to use against diseases before actual symptoms are manifest.

This herb is high in Vitamins C and B-complex. It contains sodium, silicon, phosphorus, and some iron, zinc, sulphur, nickel, tin, aluminum and beryllium.

Angina	HEART CONDITION
ANTISEPTIC	HEART PALPITATION
ARTERIOSCLEROSIS	HIGH BLOOD PRESSURE
(PREVENTS)	HYPOGLYCEMIA
Arthritis	Insomnia
CARDIAC SYMPTOMS	Kidney trouble
Congestive heart failure	LOW BLOOD PRESSURE
Dropsy	Miscarriage
ENLARGED HEART	Rheumatism, inflammatory
HARDENING OF THE	Throat, sore
ARTERIES	

HOPS (häps)
(Humulus lupulus)
Parts used: Flower

Hops is recognized for its remarkable sedative powers. It is known as one of the best nervines in the herb kingdom. It is strong but safe to use. Culpeper says, "It opens obstructions of the liver and spleen, cleanses the blood, loosens the belly, cleanses the veins from gravel and provokes urine." Hops contains appetizing and tonic properties as well as sedative properties and acts as a nervine in overcoming insomnia. It acts as a stimulant to the glands and muscles of the stomach and at the same time calms the hyperexcitability to the gastric nerves. It has a relaxing influence upon the liver and gall duct and is also a laxative to the bowels. Its main uses are to alleviate nervous tension and promote restful sleep.

Hops is rich in the vitamin B-complex. It contains magnesium, zinc, copper, traces of iodine, manganese, iron, sodium, lead, fluorine, and chlorine.

APPETITE STIMULANT
Blood cleanser
BRONCHITIS
Bruises
Cramps, abdominal
DELIRIUM
DIGESTION
Dizziness
Earache
Female problems
Fevers, high
Gallstones
HEADACHES
HYPERACTIVITY
Hysteria

INSOMNIA
Itching
Jaundice
Kidney stones
NERVOUSNESS
Neuralgia
PAIN
SEXUAL DESIRES,
 EXCESSIVE
Skin irritations
Toothache
Venereal disease
Water retention
Whooping cough
Worms

HOREHOUND (hôr'-hound)
(Marrubium vulgare)
Parts used: The Herb

Horehound is excellent in childrens' coughs, croups and colds. Its expectorant properties assists in loosening tough phlegm from the chest. It will sustain the vocal cords in congestion and hoarseness. Horehound promotes the healing of wounds and stimulates bile secretions. Warm infusion will relieve the hyperemic conditions of the lungs and congestion by promoting an outward flow of blood. It acts as a tonic to the respiratory organs and to the stomach, but in large doses, it acts as a laxative. Some herbalists have recommended it to promote delayed menstruation. It has been recommended for herpes simplex, eruptions, eczema and shingles by applying the dried herb topically.

It contains vitamins A, E, C, and F. It also contains B-complex, iron, potassium, and sulphur.

ASTHMA	Jaundice
Bronchitis	Laxative, mild
Catarrh	LUNGS
COLDS	Menstruation (produces)
COUGHS	PHLEGM
CROUP	Shingles, external
Earaches, external	STOMACH TONIC
Eczema, external	Sweating (promotes)
Fevers	RESPIRATORY ORGANS
Glands (stimulates)	Tonic
HOARSENESS	Typhoid fever
HYSTERIA	Worms (expel)
Infectious diseases	Wounds

HORSERADISH   (hôrs'-răd-ĭsh)
(Cochlearia armoracia)
Parts used: Root

Horseradish has an antibiotic action which is recommended for respiratory and urinary infections. It is a strong stimulant for the system and has been used internally to clear the nasal passages and cleans the system of infection. It has been used as a stimulant for digestion, metabolism and kidney function.

It is rich in vitamins C, B_1, sulphur, and potassium. It also contains vitamins A, P, B-complex, some calcium, phosphorus, iron and sodium.

APPETITE STIMULANT
Arthritis, external
Asthma
Bronchitis
CATARRH
CIRCULATION
Congestion
COUGH
DROPSY
Gout
Jaundice
Kidney

Mucous membrane
Neuralgia, external
Palsy
Rheumatism
SINUS PROBLEMS
Skin
TUMORS, SKIN AND IN-
TERNAL
Water retention
WORMS (EXPEL)
Wounds, septic

HORSETAIL or SHAVEGRASS (hôrs'-tāl')
(Equisetum arvense)
Parts used: The Herb

Horsetail or Shavegrass is used in urinary tract disorders, especially lower tract infections. Horsetail aids in coagulation and helps decrease bleeding. The most important ingredient is silicic acid which helps aid the circulation. Research has shown that fractured bones will heal much faster when horsetail is taken. Decoction applied externally will stop bleeding of wounds and heal them, and is used as a mouth-wash for mouth infections. Bathing in herbs accelerates the metabolic rate through the skin and makes them especially effective for circulation troubles, swelling of broken bones, chilblains. Also, pain of rheumatic diseases and gout is relieved.

It is rich in silicon and selenium. It contains vitamin E, pantothenic acid, PABA, copper, manganese, some sodium, cobalt, iron, and iodine.

BLADDER PROBLEMS
BLEEDING, INTERNAL
CIRCULATION   PROB-
LEMS
Dropsy

Fevers
GLANDULAR DISORDERS
Kidney problems
Liver, overactive
Menstruation, excess

NAILS, BRITTLE   Tuberculosis, pulmonary
Nervous tension   URINARY ULCERS
NOSE BLEEDS   URINATION, SUPRESSED
Skin rashes

HO-SHOU-WU   (hō-shoō-woō')
(Polygonum multiflorum)
Parts used: Root

Ho-Shou-Wu has a toning effect on the liver and kidneys.
It helps the nervous system. It can be used as a tonic for the
endocrine glands. It is said to improve health, stamina, and
resistance to diseases.

It is a member of the Smartweed family, of which Knot-
weed, Bistort and Buckwheat are most familiar to Americans.

Ho-Shou-Wu in China compares with those of Golden Seal
in the United States, or Chamomile in Germany. The properties
are also comparable with Ginseng.

It is useful for conditions of premature graying of hair,
backache, aches and pains of the knee joint, neurasthenia, and
traumatic bruises.

Anemia   Insomnia
Backache   Kidneys
Blood, strengthens   Knee (pains and ligaments)
Bones   Liver weakness
Bruises   Menstrual problems
Cancer   MUSCLES
Constipation   NERVES
Diabetes   Piles
Diarrhea   Scrofula
FERTILITY   Spleen weakness
Fever   Tumors
HAIR, PREMATURE   Vertigo
   GRAYING
Hypoglycemia

HYDRANGEA   (hī-drān-ja)
(Hydrangea arborescens)
Parts used: Leaves and Root

Hydrangea is called a remarkable herb. It contains curative principles second to none in nature. It contains alkaloids that act like cortisone and has the same cleansing power of chaparral. It is useful for preventing gravel deposits to form. It is known as a remedy for gravel and helps relieve the pain when the formations pass through the ureters from the kidneys to the bladder.

Hydrangea contains calcium, potassium, sodium, sulphur, phosphorus, iron, and magnesium.

Arteriosclerosis	GOUT
ARTHRITIS	Kidney problems
Backaches	KIDNEY STONES
BLADDER INFECTIONS	Pain
Calculi	Renal irritations
GALLSTONES	RHEUMATISM
GONORRHEA	URINARY PROBLEMS

HYSSOP   (hĭs'-ap)
(Hyssopus officinalis)
Parts used: Leaves

Hyssop is used in lung ailments. It is good for fevers to help produce sweating. Research has found that the mold that produces penicillin grows on hyssop leaves, and therefore helps the healing process. It contains essential hormone oil to build resistance to infectious diseases. Hyssop is usually mixed with other herbs for the best results. The leaves can be applied on wounds to help infections and help aid in healing. It has been used for poor digestion, breast and lung problems, cough from colds and nose and throat infections. It is useful for mucus congestion in the intestines.

Asthma
Blood pressure
Bronchitis
Bruises, external
CATARRH, CHRONIC
Colds
CONGESTION
COUGHS, IRRITABLE
Cuts, external
Dropsy
Ear ailments
Epilepsy
Fevers
Hoarseness

Intestines (mucus)
Jaundice
Kidney problems
Lice, external
Liver problems
LUNG AILMENTS
PHLEGM, HARD
Rheumatism (muscular, external)
Spleen problems
THROAT, SORE
Tonic
WHEEZING
WORMS

ICELAND MOSS (ī-sland mȏs)
(Cetraria islandica)
Parts used: The Herb

Iceland Moss has been known for centuries as a cure for all kinds of chest ailments. It is used to nourish weakly children, invalids and aged persons. This herb is not a moss but a lichen. It was believed to cure tuberculosis.

Iceland Moss has the same properties as Irish Moss, so the vitamin and mineral content is probably about the same. It is high in iodine, calcium, potassium and phosphorus.

ANEMIA
BRONCHITIS
CATARRH
CONGESTION
COUGHS
Diarrhea
DIGESTIVE TROUBLES

Dysentery
Fevers
Gastritis
Hoarseness
Lactation
LUNG PROBLEMS
Tuberculosis

IRISH MOSS (ĭ-rĭsh mŏs)
(Chondrus crispus)
Parts used: The Whole Plant

Irish Moss is a very useful herb when recovering from illness, because of its high content of nutrients. It has a high mucilage content, which makes it soothing to inflamed tissues and lung and kidney problems. It has been used externally to soften skin and prevent wrinkles. It purifies and strengthens the cellular structure and vital fluids of the system. The iodine contained in its small and usable quantities contributes to the glandular system. It has a beneficial effect on all the functions of the body in addition to its use as an aid to the mucous membranes.

Irish Moss contains vitamins A, D, E, F, and K. It is high in iodine, calcium and sodium. It contains some phosphorus, potassium and sulphur. This herb contains 15 elements of 18 composing the human body.

Bladder problems	Joints, swollen
BRONCHITIS	LUNG PROBLEMS
Cancer	THYROID
Halitosis (bad breath)	Tuberculosis
Intestinal problems	Tumors
GLANDS	Ulcers, peptic
GOITER	Varicose veins

JOJOBA (yō-yō-bä)
(Simmondsia chinensis)
Parts used: Oil

Jojoba oil from the seed has been used by Indians to promote hair growth and relieve skin problems since before Columbus discovered America. Scientists have found that deposits of sebum tends to collect around hair follicles, solidify and cause dandruff, hair loss and scalp disorders. Jojoba oil removes the embedded sebum and makes the scalp less acidic.

Jojoba contains B-complex, vitamin E, silicon, chromium and is very high in iodine. It also has copper and zinc.

Abrasions	Mouth sores
Acne (vulgaris)	Pimples
Athletes foot	PSORIASIS
CHAPPED SKIN	SCALP, DRY
Cuts	Seborrhea
DANDRUFF	SKIN, DRY
Eczema	Warts
HAIR LOSS	Wrinkles

JUNIPER   (jōō'-na-par)
(Juniperis species)
Parts used: Berries

Juniper is used in cases where uric acid is being retained in the system. It is an excellent disease preventative. In ancient Europe the scent of Juniper was believed to ward off the plague. It is high in natural insulin. It has the ability to restore the pancreas where there has been no permanent damage. It is excellent for infections.

Juniper is high in vitamin C. It contains sulphur, copper, and a high content of cobalt, a trace of tin and aluminum.

Ague	DROPSY
BLEEDING	Gas
Bladder problems	Gonorrhea
Catarrhal inflammations	Gums, bleeding
COLDS	INFECTIONS
Colic	Insect bites, poisonous
Coughs	KIDNEY INFECTIONS
Convulsions	Leucorrhea
Cramps	Menstruation (regulates)
Diabetes	PANCREAS

Piles
Snakebites
Sores
Tuberculosis
Typhoid fever

URIC ACID, BUILD UP
URINARY DISORDERS
WATER RETENTION
Worms

KELP   (kĕlp)
(Fucus versiculosus)
Parts used: The Whole Plant

Kelp is a good promoter of glandular health. It controls the thyroid and regulates the metabolism which helps digest food. Kelp has the reputation of speeding up the burning of excess calories by controlling the body's metabolism and is helpful in the nourishment of the body with its ability to stimulate metabolism. It contains all of the minerals considered vital to health. It even contains a small amount of lecithin. Kelp has a beneficial effect on many disorders of the body. It is called a sustainer to the nervous system and the brain, helping the brain to function normally. It is essential during pregnancy.

Kelp contains nearly 30 minerals. It is rich in iodine, calcium, sulphur and silicon. It also contains phosphorus, iron, sodium, potassium, magnesium, chlorine, copper, zinc and manganese. It has a small amount of barium, boron, chromium, lithium, nickel, silver, titanium, vanadium, aluminum, strontium, bismuth, chlorine, cobalt, gallium, tin and zirconium. Kelp is rich in B-complex vitamins. It contains vitamin A, C, E and G. It also contains anti-sterility vitamin S, and it has anti-hemmorhage vitamin K.

ADRENAL GLANDS
ARTERIES (CLEANS)
Asthma
COLITIS
COMPLEXION
Constipation
Diabetes

Digestion, poor
ECZEMA
FINGERNAILS
Gallbladder
Gas
GOITER
Headaches

High blood pressure
Kidneys
Morning sickness
Nervous disorder
Neuritis
OBESITY
Pancreas
PITUITARY GLAND

Prostate (tones)
Skin
THYROID GLAND
Uterus, weak
Vitality, low
Water retention
Wrinkles

LADY'S SLIPPER   (lā'-dies slĭp'-ar)
(Cypripedium pubescens)
Parts used: Root

Lady's Slipper acts as a tonic for the exhausted nervous system. It has a calming effect on the body and mind. It is said to be the most excellent and safest nervine in the plant kingdom. It can be used for weakly and nervous children, especially for symptoms of twitching muscles. Its action is slow, yet it works on the entire nervous system. It is an excellent pain reliever. It acts primarily on the medulla, helping to regulate breathing, sweating, saliva and heart functions.

It contains the B complex vitamins.

Abdominal pain
After pains
CHOREA
Colic
Cramps
Cystic Fibrosis
Epilepsy
Headaches, nervous
HYSTERIA

INSOMNIA
Muscle spasms
NERVOUSNESS
Neuralgia
PAIN
RESTLESSNESS
Tremors
Typhoid fever

LEMON GRASS   (lem'-en gras)
(Cymbopogon citratus)
Parts used: Leaves

Lemon Grass has a mild effect, which makes it an excellent remedy for people under stress and for women suffering from cramps, headaches and dizziness. It has been highly recommended for feverish colds. It has an astringent or tightening action on the tissues of the body which helps to stop or slow discharge from mucous membranes. It is very useful for infants and children's diseases. It has been used an an anti-fever tea for colds, flu and fevers. It is very high in vitamin A and vitamin C.

Bladder	Insect Bites
Boils (warm poultice)	Kidneys
COLDS	Liver
Colic	Menstruation, suppressed
DIGESTION	Nausea
FEVERS	Nervousness
Gas	Spleen
Headaches	Vomiting
High blood pressure	

LICORICE (lĭk'-ar-ĭsh)
(Glycyrrhiza glabra)
Parts used: Root

Licorice is a source of the female hormone estrogen. It is a very important herb for female complaints. Licorice works as a stimulant on the adrenal glands. It contains glycosides which can chemically purge excess fluid from the lungs, throat and body. It is well known for coughs and chest complaints. It is an important herb when recovering from illness, for it will supply necessary energy to the system. It works as a laxative and helps in inflammation of the intestinal tract and relieves ulcer conditions. It has a stimulating action and helps counteract stress.

It contains vitamin E, phosphorus, B-complex, biotin, niacin, and pantothenic acid. It also contains lecithin, manganese, iodine, chromium, and zinc.

Adrenal exhaustion	Age spots
ADDISON'S DISEASE	Arteriosclerosis

Arthritis	FEMALE COMPLAINTS
BLOOD CLEANSER	Fevers
Bronchial congestion	Flu
Circulation	Heart (strengthens)
COLDS	HOARSENESS
Constipation	HYPOGLYCEMIA
COUGH	Impotency
Cushing's disease	Liver
Dropsy	LUNG PROBLEMS
DRUG WITHDRAWAL	PHLEGM (EXPELS)
Emphysema	THROAT (SORE)
Endurance	TONIC
ENERGY	Ulcers

LOBELIA   (lō-bē′-lē-a, bēlya)
(Lobelia inflata)
Parts used: The Herb

Lobelia is a valuable herb. It is well known for removing obstructions from any part of the system. Lobelia is the most powerful relaxant in the herb kingdom, and modern use has shown that it has no harmful effects. Dr. Thomson said that there is no herb more powerful in removing disease and promoting health than Lobelia. It has healing powers with the ability to remove congestion within the body, especially the blood vessels. It has a genuine effect on the whole system. Lobelia is a special herb for bronchial spasms. Lobelia was used externally in a poultice with Slippery Elm and a little soap was useful in bringing abscesses or boils to a head.

Lobelia contains sulphur, iron, cobalt, selenium, sodium, copper, and lead.

Allergies	Childhood diseases
ARTHRITIS, (TINCTURE)	Circulation
ASTHMA	COLDS
Blood poisoning	Colic
BRONCHITIS	CONGESTION
CATARRH	Constipation

CONVULSIONS	Palsy
COUGH	Pleurisy
Cramps	PNEUMONIA
CROUP, (TINCTURE)	Poison ivy and oak
EARACHE, (TINCTURE)	Rheumatism
EAR INFECTIONS	Rabies
Eczema	Ringworm, (tincture)
EPILEPSY	Scarlet fever
Female problems	Shock
FEVERS	SPASMS
FOOD POISONING	Syphilis
Headache	Teeth
Heart	Tetanus
Hepatitis	Tonsillitis
Hydrophobia	Toothaches
LOCK JAW, (TINCTURE)	Vomiting, (small doses)
LUNG PROBLEMS	WHOOPING COUGH
MISCARRIAGE	WORMS
NERVOUSNESS	Wounds
PAIN	

MANDRAKE (American) (măn'-drāk')
(Podophyllum peltatum)
Parts used: Root

Mandrake (American) is a very strong glandular stimulant. It is used for treatment of chronic liver diseases, skin problems, bile flow, digestion and eliminating obstructions. Mandrake is often combined with supporting herbs to regulate liver and bowels, for uterine disorders and intermittent fevers. It is being used as a natural plant cure for cancer in experiments to destroy cancer cells in test animals. It is a powerful herb and should be used with caution. It should not be used during pregnancy. Mandrake has been said to be a rejuvenator as well as a cure for sterile women.

Asthma	CONSTIPATION
BOWELS, LOWER	Diarrhea
CANCER	Dropsy

FEVERS	Rheumatism
Gallstones	Scrofula
Hay fever	Skin problems
Headaches	Syphilis
INDIGESTION	Typhoid fever
Jaundice	Vomiting
Lead poisoning	Warts
LIVER PROBLEMS	Whooping Cough
Nervousness	WORMS
Pain, chronic	

MARIGOLD   (mār'-a-gōld')
(Calendula officinalis)
Parts used: The Herb

Marigold is very useful herb to keep on hand as a first aid remedy. It has been used in the ears to relieve earaches or as a tea for acute ailments, especially for fevers. It is also useful for bleeding hemorrhoids. It is effective as a tincture when applied to bruises, sprains, muscle spasms, and ulcers. It has been used as a snuff to discharge mucus from the nose. It is said by some herbalists to be excellent for the heart and for circulation. It has an excellent effect on old or badly healed scars.

Marigold is high in phosphorus and contains vitamins A and C.

Amenorrhea	EYE INFECTIONS
Anemia	Fevers
Blood cleansers	Hemorrhoids
Bronchitis	Hepatitis
BRUISES, EXTERNAL	Jaundice
Cancer	SKIN DISEASES
Colitis	TOOTHACHE
Cramps	Ulcers
CUTS, EXTERNAL	Varicose veins
Diarrhea	Worms (expels)
Ear infections	Wounds

MARJORAM (mār-jar-am)
(Origanum vulgare)
Parts used: The Herb

Marjoram has tonic, stimulant and carminative properties. Therefore, it is useful in asthma, coughs and various spasmodic afflictions. One custom is to give warm infusion of Marjoram at the onset of measles. It produces a gentle perspiration and brings out the eruption. It helps to strengthen stomach and intestines and is used as an antidote for narcotic poisons, convulsions and dropsy.

Marjoram contains vitamins A and C, niacin, some thiamine, riboflavin, and vitamin B_{12}. Also it contains calcium potassium, magnesium, phosphorus, some iron, sodium, zinc, and silicon.

Asthma
Bedwetting
COLIC
Convulsions
COUGHS, VIOLENT
CRAMPS, ABDOMINAL
Diarrhea
Dropsy
Fevers
GAS
Gastritis
HEADACHES, NERVOUS

INDIGESTION
Measles (regulates)
Narcotic poisoning
Nightmares
Nausea
Neuralgia
RESPIRATORY
   PROBLEMS
Seasickness
Toothaches (oil)
Tuberculosis
Water retention
Whooping cough

MARSHMALLOW
(Althaea officinalis)
Parts used: Root

(märsh'-mĕl'-ō, măl'-ō)

Marshmallow contains mucilage which helps aid the expectorant influence of difficult phlegm and helps relax the bronchial tubes while soothing and healing. It is valuable for all lung ailments. It is especially good for asthma and helps remove mucus from the lungs. It heals inflammation and prevents gangrene and other infections. It is a great healing herb. It is a powerful anti-inflammatory and anti-irritant for the joint and the gastrointestinal tract. Marshmallow is also protective and healing in the irritations associated with diarrhea and dysentery. Used externally as a poultice with cayenne, it can be used to treat blood poisoning, gangrene, burns, bruises, and wounds.

It contains 286,000 units of vitamin A per pound. It is very high in calcium, and marshmallow is extremely rich in zinc. It also contains iron, sodium, iodine, B-complex, and pantothenic acid.

ASTHMA	Glands
BLEEDING, URINARY	Gravel
BOILS	Intestines
Breast problems	KIDNEYS
BRONCHIAL INFECTIONS	Lactation
Burns (acid or fire)	Liver problems
Catarrh	LUNG CONGESTION
Constipation	Mucous membrane
Cough, dry	Skin
Diabetes	Stomach problems
Diarrhea	Throat, sore
Dysentery	Urinary infections
EMPHYSEMA	WHOOPING COUGH
Eyes, sore	WOUNDS, INFECTED

MILK THISTLE (milk-this' tle)
(Silybum marianum)
Part Used: Seeds

Milk Thistle was used centuries ago by the Romans for restoring impaired liver function. It is currently being used in Europe to restore as well as protect the liver. In Germany it is used for the treatment of liver diseases including amanita mushroom poisoning. This mushroom is often fatal, destroying liver cells. Milk Thistle can block the damage and regenerate the liver cells.

Milk Thistle is an antioxidant to protect against free radical scavengers. It has an overall effect on the whole body because of the function of the liver in protecting the immune system. This herb plays a major role in protecting, rejuvenating and restoring liver function. It helps prevent plaque buildup and hardening of the arteries. Its action is to protect the liver and prevent sickness.

Milk Thistle is rich in bioflavonoids which act in the body to increase membrane strength and reduce membrane permeability. It stimulates protein synthesis, while accelerating the process of liver regeneration in damaged tissues.

Alcoholism	Heartburn
Appetite Stimulant	Hepatitis
Boils	Indigestion
Chemotherapy (protects against)	Liver Damage
Cirrhosis	Radiation
Depression	Skin Diseases
Fatty Deposits	Toxic Poisons
Gas	

MISTLETOE   (mis-el-tō)
(Phoradendron flavescens)
Parts used: The Herb

Mistletoe acts on the circulatory system. It increases then lowers blood pressure. Mistletoe can also constrict blood vessels and stimulate the heart beat. Hippocrates claimed that Mistletoe was an excellent remedy for the spleen. Some modern European physicians believe that treating the spleen may be beneficial in cases of epilepsy. Mistletoe is one of the best natural tranquilizers and is not habit forming. It is beneficial in migraine headaches. Used in any condition where there is a weakness or disordered state of the nervous system, Mistletoe is a useful herb. It will quiet and soothe the nerves and reduce cerebral activity.

Mistletoe contains vitamin B_{12}, calcium, sodium, magnesium, potassium, iron, cobalt, iodine, copper, and cadmium.

Arteriosclerosis
Arthritis
Asthma
Bed wetting
Blood cleanser
Cholera
CHOREA
CIRCULATION (STIMU-
   LATES)
CONVULSIONS
Delirium
EPILEPSY
Gall bladder
Heart problems

HEMORRHAGES,
   INTERNAL
HIGH BLOOD PRESSURE
Hypertension
Hypoglycemia
Hysteria
Mental disturbance
MENSTRUATION
Migraine headaches
NERVOUSNESS
Neuralgia
Rheumatism
SPLEEN
Tonic
Tumors

MULLEIN (mul'-en)
(Verbascum thapsus)
Parts used: Leaves

Mullein is called a natural wonder herb with narcotic properties, without being habit forming or poisonous. Mullein is a great pain killer and helps induce sleep. It has a calming effect on all inflamed and irritated nerves. This is why it works so well in controlling coughs, cramps and spasms. It has the ability to loosen mucus and move it out of the body. It is valuable for all lung problems because it nourishes as well as strengthens. The crushed fresh flowers have been used to remove warts. The tea has been used for dropsy, sinusitis, and swollen joints. The hot tea helps when applied to mumps, tumors, sore throat, and tonsillitis.

Mullein is high in iron, magnesium, potassium and sulphur. It contains vitamins A, D, and B-complex.

ASTHMA
BLEEDING (BOWEL AND
  LUNGS)
Bowel complaints
BRONCHITIS
Bruises
Colds
COUGHS
Cramps
CROUP
Diaper rash
DIARRHEA
Dropsy
DYSENTERY
EARACHES (OIL)
Female problems
Gas

Glands, cleans
Hay fever
Hemorrhage
Hemorrhoids
Hoarseness
INSOMNIA
LYMPHATIC SYSTEM
Lung problems
NERVOUSNESS
PAIN (RELIEVES)
PLEURISY
Pneumonia
SINUS CONGESTION
Sores
TUBERCULOSIS
Venereal diseases
Wounds

MUSTARD   (mus'-terd)
(Sinapis alba)
Parts used: Seeds

Mustard is a strong stimulating herb. The seeds are the part
that is used. They promote appetite and stimulate the gastrate
mucous membrane which helps in digestion. An infusion of the
seed stimulates the urine and helps in delayed menstruation. It is
a valuable emetic for narcotic poisoning because it empties the
stomach without depression of the system. Mustard is used
externally as a plaster or poultice. It is used as a plaster for sore,
stiff muscles to loosen them up and carry away the toxins that
cause the muscles to tighten.

Mustard is an excellent source of calcium, phosphorus and
potassium. It contains vitamins A, B_1, B_2, B_{12} and C. It also
contains sulphur, iron, cobalt and traces of manganese and
iodine.

INTERNAL:

Appetite stimulant
Bad breath
Blood purifier
Bronchitis
Emphysema
GAS
Hiccoughs
INDIGESTION
Pleurisy
Snake bites
Sore throat

EXTERNAL:

Arthritis
Feet (sore)
Fever
Kidneys
LIVER
LUNGS
Pneumonia
Sprains

MYRRH   (mʉr)
(Balsamodendron myrrha)
Parts used: Resin

Myrrh is a powerful antiseptic on the mucous membranes. It has been said that Myrrh is a remedy second only to echinacea. It is valuable as a cleansing and healing agent to the stomach and colon for it helps sooth inflammation and speeds the healing process. The essential oils contain antiseptic properties and when used as a tincture mixed with water it is excellent as a gargle for sore throat. It has been used with golden seal to make a healing antiseptic salve. Myrrh gives vitality and strength to the digestive system. It helps in waste elimination.

Abrasions	Indigestion
Asthma	LUNG DISEASES
BAD BREATH	Menstrual problems
Bed sores	MOUTH SORES
BRONCHITIS	Nipples, sore
CATARRH, CHRONIC	Piles
COLON (CLEANS)	Pimples
Coughs	Scarlet fever
Cuts	Sinus problems
Diarrhea, chronic	SKIN SORES
Eczema	STOMACH (CLEANS)
Gas	THROAT, SORE
GUMS	Tuberculosis
HEMORRHOIDS	Ulcers
Herpes	Wounds

NETTLE   (net'-le)
(Urtica dioica)
Parts used: Leaves

Nettle is one of the most useful of all plants according to folks of the old world in Europe. They have learned this from centuries of experience. It has been said that "the sting of the Nettle is but nothing compared to the pains that it heals." (Lelord Kordels', *Natural Folk Remedies*) The plant contains alkaloids that neutralize uric acid which help in rheumatism. It is rich in iron which is vital in circulation and helpful in high blood pressure. The tannin in the root has been used as an astringent enema to shrink hemorrhoids and reduce excess menstrual flow.

Nettle is so rich in chlorophyll that the English used it to make the green dye used in World War II as camouflage paint. It is rich in iron, silicon, and potassium. It is rich in vitamins A and C. It contains a high content of protein. It also contains vitamins E, F and P, calcium, sulphur, sodium, copper, manganese, chromium and zinc. It contains first-class calcium and vitamin D.

Anemia
Asthma
BLEEDING, INTERNAL
BLEEDING, EXTERNAL
BLOOD PURIFIER
BRONCHITIS
CATARRHAL
  CONDITIONS
Circulation, poor
DIARRHEA
DYSENTERY
Eczema

Hemorrhoids
HIGH BLOOD PRESSURE
Hives
Kidneys, inflamed
Menstruation, excess
Mouth sores
Nosebleeds
Piles, bleeding
RHEUMATISM
Skin ailments
Vaginitis

OATSTRAW   (ōt-strò)
(*Avena sativa*)
Parts used: Stems

Oatstraw is a powerful stimulant and is rich in body-building materials. In homoeopathy a tincture is made from the fresh flowering plant and is used in arthritis, rheumatism, paralysis, liver infections and skin diseases. Hot oatstraw compresses applied to painful areas, when in pain, from kidney stone attacks has brought relief. Oatstraw has many elements that have antiseptic properties and is said to be a natural preventative for contagious diseases when taken frequently as a food.

Oatstraw is high in silicon and rich in calcium. It contains phosphorus and vitamins A, B_1, B_2 and E.

Arthritis
BED WETTING
Bladder
Boils
Bones, brittle
Bursitis
Constipation
Eyes
Gall bladder
Gout
INDIGESTION

INSOMNIA
HEART (STRENGTHENS)
Kidneys
Liver
Lungs
NERVES
Pancreas
Paralysis
Rheumatism
URINARY ORGANS
Wounds

OREGON GRAPE   (ōr'-i-gun grāp)
(*Berberis aquifolium*)
Parts used: Rhizome and Root

Oregon Grape is well known for the treatment of skin diseases due to toxins in the blood. It stimulates the action on the

44

liver and is one of the best blood cleansers. It is a mild stimulant on the thyroid functions. Oregon Grape aids in the assimilation of nutrients, with its stimulating and purifying properties. It is a tonic for all the glands. It can be substituted for golden seal.

Oregon Grape contains minerals such as manganese, silicon, sodium, copper, and zinc.

ACNE
APPETITE (INCREASES)
Arthritis, rheumatoid
BLOOD CONDITIONS
Bowels
Bronchitis
Constipation, chronic
DIGESTION (PROMOTES)
ECZEMA
Hepatitis
Herpes
JAUNDICE
Kidneys
Leucorrhea
LIVER
Lymph glands
PSORIASIS
Rheumatism
Scrofula
SKIN DISEASES
STAPH INFECTION
Strength (increases)
Syphilis
Uterine diseases
Vaginitis (douche)

PAPAYA   (pa-pī-a)
(Carica papaya)
Parts used: Fruit

Papaya contains papain, an enzyme that breaks down protein food to a digestible state. The juice has been used to dissolve corns, warts and pimples. Ulcerated skin and open wounds have been treated by wrapping fresh papaya leaves around them. Papaya has been used to heal ulcers and other internal bleeding. It has been used for cleaning discharges of the middle ear. The seeds are given with honey and are used for expelling worms, bleeding piles and enlargement of the liver and spleen. The paste of the seeds is used and applied to skin diseases like ringworm. It is valued as a blood clotting agent and has been used to stop bleeding. Papaya is a fruit to use after meals to help digest the food. Papaya contains vitamins B, D, E, G, K, and C. It also contains calcium, iron, phosphorus and potassium. It is rich in sodium, magnesium, and vitamin A.

Allergies	GAS
Blood clotting	Hemorrhage
COLON	INSECT BITES
Burns	INTESTINAL TRACT
Constipation	Sores
DIGESTION	Stomach problems
Diarrhea, chronic	Worms
Freckles (juice)	Wounds

PARSLEY (pär-slē)
(Petroselinum sativum)
Parts used: Leaves

Parsley should be used as a preventative herb. It is so nutritious that it increases resistance to infections and diseases. The roots or leaves are very good for all liver and spleen problems when jaundice and venereal diseases are present. Fresh juice has helped in conjunctivitis and blepharitis, an inflammation of the eyelid. It has a tonic effect on the entire urinary system. It has been used as a cancer preventative. Parsley should not be used during pregnancy, it could bring on labor pains. It will dry up mother's milk after birth.

Parsley is high in vitamin B and potassium. It is said to contain a substance in which cancerous cells cannot multiply. It is rich in iron, chlorophyll, and vitamins A and C. Parsley increases iron content in the blood. It contains some sodium, copper, thiamine and riboflavin. It also contains some silicon, sulphur, calcium and cobalt.

Allergies	Hay fever
Arthritis	JAUNDICE
Asthma	KIDNEY INFLAMMATION
BLADDER INFECTIONS	Liver
BLOOD BUILDER	Lumbago
BLOOD CLEANSER	Menstruation (promotes)
Blood pressure (low)	Pituitary
Breath (bad)	Prostate
Cancer	Rheumatism
Coughs	Sciatica
Digestion (aids)	Thyroid
DROPSY	Tumors
Eyes	URINE RETENTION
GALLSTONES	Varicose veins
Gonorrhea	Venereal diseases
Gout	

PASSION FLOWER   (pa'-shun flou'-er)
(Passiflora incarnata)
Parts used: The Herb

Passion Flower is used in Italy to treat hyperactive children, while in Yucatan it is used for insomnia, hysteria and convulsions in children. This herb is one that doctors should recommend to patients who want to wean themselves from synthetic sleeping pills and tranquilizers. It is quieting and soothing to the nervous system. It does not bring depression nor disorientation. One doctor says that Passion Flower kills a form of bacteria that causes eye irritations. Therefore, it is good for inflamed eyes and dimness of vision. He says in some cases it surpasses eyebright for inflamed eyes and dimness of vision. It is a good herb for nervousness such as unrest, agitation and exhaustion. It is helpful in contolling convulsions, especially in young children.

Asthma, spasmodic	High blood pressure
Convulsions	Hysteria
Diarrhea	INSOMNIA
Dysentery	MENOPAUSE
Epilepsy	Menstruation, painful
EYE INFECTION	Muscle spasms
Eye strain	Nervous breakdown
EYE TENSION	Neuralgia
FEVERS	Pain
Headaches	Vision (dimness)

PEACH (pēch)
(Prunus persica)
Parts used: Bark and Leaves

Peach contains curative powers. The powdered dried leaves have been used to heal sores and wounds. In *Back to Eden*, the leaves and bark have been referred to as a substitute for quinine. It contains strengthening powers for the nervous system. It stimulates the flow of urine, has mild sedative properties and is useful for chronic bronchitis and chest complaints because of its expectorant properties.

BLADDER	Nervousness
BRONCHITIS, CHRONIC	Sores
CONGESTION, CHEST	Stomach problems
Constipation	Uterine problems
Insomnia	WATER RETENTION
Jaundice	Whooping cough
Morning sickness	WORMS
Mucus	Wounds
NAUSEA	

PENNYROYAL   (pen'-ē-roi-al)
(Hedeoma Pulegioides)
Parts used: The Herb

Pennyroyal contains the volatile oil which works in the stomach to remove gas. It can be taken as a tea or used as a hot footbath a few days before menstruation is due to help a suppressed flow. This is also useful for colds. It has a strong minty smell and is used externally to repel insects such as fleas, flies and mosquitos. It has been used to induce abortions, but it can cause serious problems. It can be used just before delivery.

Pennyroyal contains minerals such as lead and sodium.

Abdominal cramps	LUNG INFECTIONS
Catarrh	Measles
BRONCHITIS	MENSTRUATION (PROM-
CHILDBIRTH	OTES)
COLDS	Mucus
COLIC	Nausea
Convulsions	NERVOUSNESS
Coughs	Phlegm (expels)
CRAMPS	Pleurisy
Delirium	Pneumonia
Earache	Smallpox
FEMALE PROBLEMS	Sunstroke
FEVERS	SWEATING (INDUCES)
Flu	Toothache
GAS	Tuberculosis
Gout	Ulcers
Headaches, migraine	Uterus
Leprosy	Vertigo

PEPPERMINT   (pēp-ar-mint')
(Mentha piperita)
Parts used: Leaves

Peppermint has a warming oil that is as effective as a nerve stimulant. The oil brings oxygen into the blood steam. This herb cleans and strengthens the entire body. Peppermint also acts as a sedative on the stomach and helps strengthen the bowels. It is useful for bowel problems, convulsions and spasms in children. It works on the salivary glands to help as an aid in digestion. Peppermint is an herb that is good for many remedies and is useful to have in the house. It is very soothing to the system as well as strengthening for the heart muscles. It is useful in chills and colds. It can be used for many ailments.

Peppermint contains vitamins A and C. It also contains magnesium, potassium, inositol, niacin, copper, iodine, silicon, iron and sulphur.

APPETITE
Bowel spasms
Chills
Cholera
COLDS
COLIC
Constipation
Convulsions
Cramps, stomach
Depression, mental
DIGESTION
Dizziness
Fainting
FEVER
Flu
GAS
HEADACHES

Heart
HEARTBURN
Hysteria
Insomnia
Measles
Menstruation pain
Morning sickness
Mouthwash
Nausea
Nerves
Neuralgia
Nightmares
Seasickness
SHOCK
Stomach spasms
Vomiting

PERIWINKLE (pēri-wing'-kal)
(Vinca major; Vinca minor)
Parts used: The Herb, Leaves

Periwinkle has been reported by British physicians to contain a substance called vinblastine sulphate. This substance has shown promising results for choriocarcinoma and Hodgkin's disease. It is under further research for other types of cancer such as lung cancer. Periwinkle is also considered a good binder

to stop bleeding of the nose or mouth, when chewed. It is good
for female problems.

Bleeding	Leukemia
CANCER	Mucus
Congestion	NERVOUSNESS
Constipation, chronic	Nightmares
Cramps	PILES (BLEEDING)
Dandruff, external	Skin disorders
DIABETES	Sores
Diarrhea, chronic	Toothache
Fits	ULCERS
Hemorrhages, internal	Wounds
Hysteria	

PLANTAIN   (plān'-tan)
(Plantago major)
Parts used: Leaves and Seeds

   Plantain will neutralize the stomach acids and normalize
all stomach secretions. It clears the ears of mucus. It is used for
the first stages of venereal diseases. As a tea, it is used to clear
the head of mucus. It is also known to neutralize poisons. The
leaves, when applied to a bleeding surface, will stop hemorrhaging. It is useful in treating chronic lung problems in children (as a mild tea). The fresh juice has been used in mild
stomach ulcers. The seeds are related to psyllium seeds and can
be used in the same way.
   Plantain is rich in vitamins C, K and T. It is rich in calcium,
potassium, and sulphur. There is high content of trace minerals.

BED WETTING	DIARRHEA
BLADDER INFECTIONS	Dropsy
BLOOD POISONING	Dysentery
Blood purifier	Epilepsy
Bronchitis	Eyes, sore
Burns	Fevers, intermittent
Coughs	Gas
Cuts	Hemorrhages, external

b

Hemorrhoids
Infections
Insect bites
Jaundice
KIDNEY
Leucorrhea
Menstruation, excess
NEURALGIA
Respiratory problems
Scalds

Scrofula
Skin problems
SNAKE BITES
SORES
Stings
Water retention
ULCERS
Worms
WOUNDS, CHRONIC

PLEURISY ROOT   (plōōr-a-sē rōōt)
(Asclepias tuberosa)
Parts used: Root

Pleurisy Root is effective as an expectorant. It helps to expel phlegm from bronchial and nasal passages. It is a gentle tonic for pain in the stomach, as in gas, indigestion and dysentery. It is not recommended for children. It is valuable in pleurisy, helping the pain and relieving the difficulty of breathing, and is also recommended in pulmonary catarrh.

ASTHMA, SPASMODIC
BRONCHITIS
Catarrh
Contagious diseases
Croup
DYSENTERY, ACUTE
EMPHYSEMA
FEVERS
Flu
Kidneys
LUNG PROBLEMS

Measles
Mucus
Perspiration
PLEURISY
PNEUMONIA
Poisoning
Rheumatism, acute
Scarlet fever
Tuberculosis
Typhus

POKEWEED   (pōk-wēd)
(Phytolacca americana)
Parts used: Root and Young Shoots

Pokeweed is excellent for enlarged glands (lymphatic, spleen and thyroid), hardening of the liver and reduced biliary flow. It stimulates metabolism and is a useful medication of the undernourished. It reduces inflammation, so it is useful for rheumatism, tonsillitis, laryngitis and mumps. It is used externally as a salve to treat scabies, acne and fungal infections, and as a poultice for abscesses. Pokeweed contains steroids resembling cortisone, making it useful in treating psoriasis, rheumatism, and slow healing wounds. The young shoots are used. Pokeweed has been used by the Indians as a cure for surface cancers and skin eruptions, applied as a powdered root poultice. The pioneers used the berry juice on skin cancers and wounds. Pokeweed should be used sparingly and by one trained in using herbs. It has been used as an aid in weight reduction and to stimulate a sluggish glandular system.

It contains vitamins A and C. It also has calcium, iron, and phosphorus.

ARTHRITIS	Lymphs
BLOOD PURIFIER	Mumps
Cancer	PAIN
Catarrh, chronic	Respiratory problems
GLANDS	RHEUMATISM
Goiter	Scrofula
INFLAMMATION	Skin diseases
Laryngitis	Tonsillitis
Laxative	

PRICKLY ASH   (prīk-lē ăsh)
(Xanthoxylum fraxineum)
Parts used: Bark

Prickly Ash is a stimulant herb that increases the circulation throughout the body. It is beneficial in most cases of impaired circulation such as cold extremities and joints, rheumatism and arthritis, lethargy, and wounds that are slow to heal. Prickly Ash is applied externally as a poultice to help dry up and heal wounds. The powdered bark has been chewed for relief of toothache. Prickly Ash will help increase the flow of saliva and moisten the dry tongue, which often accompanies liver malfunctions, and is useful in paralysis of the tongue and mouth.

Arthritis	Gas
Asthma	Lethargy
Blood purifier	Liver problems
Cholera	Paralysis
CIRCULATION, POOR	Rheumatism, chronic
Colic	Scrofula
Cramps	Skin diseases
Digestion, weak	SORES, MOUTH
Diarrhea	Syphilis
Dropsy	ULCERS
Female problems	WOUNDS
FEVER	

PSYLLIUM   (sil-lium)
(Plantago ovata)
Parts used: Seeds

Psyllium is considered an excellent colon and intestine cleanser. It lubricates as well as heals the intestines and colon. It does not irritate the mucous membranes of the intestines but strengthens the tissues and restores tone. It is said to be very good for auto-intoxication, which can cause many diseases, by cleansing the intestines and removing the toxins.

Colitis	Gonorrhea
COLON BLOCKAGE	Hemorrhage
CONSTIPATION	Intestinal tract
DIVERTICULITIS	Ulcers
Dysentery	Urinary tract

QUASSIA   (kwäsh'-a)
(Picrasma amara)
Parts used: Bark

Quassia is called a great healer of the sick. It is a powerful herb, and if taken to excess, is emetic, irritant and depressant, producing nausea; but if taken in small doses, it speedily cures. It is one of the best tonic herbs to help in run down systems. It is said to be a good remedy to destroy the taste for strong drink. It is said to be one of the best remedies of noxious substances in the alimentary canal resulting from the digestion process. It is beneficial to the eyes, by keeping the liver in good working condition.

It contains calcium, sodium, and potassium.

Alcoholism	FEVERS
APPETITE, STIMULANT	Pinworms, (through enema)
Constipation	Rheumatism
Dandruff, external	TONIC
DIGESTION	WORMS (EXPELS)
Dyspepsia	

QUEEN OF THE MEADOW
(kwen-of-the-mēd'-ō)
(Eupatorium purpureum)
Parts used: Leaves

Queen of the Meadow is useful for all ills of the joints, including aching or sprained back. It is used for all strains and sprains and pulled ligaments and tendons. It is well known for its usefulness in rheumatism, dropsy, kidneys and gallstones, and urinary problems. It is useful in treating water retention and joint pains caused by uric acid deposits. It has been used in chronic urinary problems, gout and cystitis.

Queen of the Meadow contains vitamins C and D.

Bladder infections
BURSITIS
Diabetes
DROPSY
GALLSTONES
Gout
Headaches
KIDNEY INFECTIONS
KIDNEY STONES

Lumbago
Nerve problems
NEURALGIA
Prostate
RHEUMATISM
RINGWORM
Typhus
URINARY PROBLEMS
WATER RETENTION

RED CLOVER   (rēd klō'-var)
(Trifolium pratense)
Parts used: Flowers

Red Clover is useful as a tonic for the nerves and as a sedative for nervous exhaustion. The Indians used the plant for sore eyes and in a salve for burns. It is useful mixed with honey and water as a cough syrup. It has been used as an antidote for cancer. It is also a very useful herb for children because of its mild alterative properties as well as a mild sedative effect. Red Clover is a valuable herb for wasting diseases (especially rickets), spasmodic affections, and whooping cough. It is also useful for delicate children to help strengthen their systems. It is good for coughs, weak chest, wheezing, bronchitis, and for lack of vitality and nervous energy.

It is a good dietary supplement to supply vitamin A. It is high in iron content. It contains B-complex, vitamins C, F, and P. It is a valued herb for its high mineral content. It contains some selenium, cobalt, nickel, manganese, sodium, and tin. Rich in magnesium, calcium, and copper.

Acne
Arthritis
Appetite
Athletes' foot poultice
BLOOD PURIFIER
Boils
BRONCHITIS

Burns
CANCER
Childhood diseases
Coughs
Eyewash
Flu
Leprosy

Liver problems
NERVES
Psoriasis
Rheumatism
Scrofula
Skin diseases
Sores
SPASMS

Syphilis
TOXINS
Tumors
Ulcers
Urinary problems
Whooping cough
Wounds, fresh

RED RASPBERRY   (red raz'-berē)
(Rubus idaeus)
Parts used: Leaves

Red Raspberry is one of the most renowned and proven herbs for women, especially during pregnancy. It contains nutrients to strengthen the uterus wall. It helps in nausea, helps prevent hemorrhage, and reduces pain and ease of childbirth. It helps reduce false labor pains so common in some pregnancies. It helps enrich colostrum found in breast milk. It is a wonderful herb for children to use for colds, diarrhea, colic and fevers in all their stages. It is good for vomiting of weakly children. It is a good remedy for dysentery and diarrhea for infants. Drinking the tea will relieve painful menstruation and aid the flow; if it is too heavy, it will decrease without abruptly stopping it. Drinking the tea after birth will help decrease uterine swelling and cut down on post partum bleeding.

Red Raspberry contains vitamins A, C, D, E, G, F, and B. It is rich in iron. It contains phosphorus, manganese and a high amount of calcium.

AFTERPAINS
BOWEL PROBLEMS
Bronchitis
Canker sores
CHILDBIRTH
Cholera
Colds
Constipation

Diabetes
DIARRHEA
Digestion
Dysentery
Eye wash
FEMALE ORGANS
FEVERS
FLU

Hemorrhoids
Lactation
Leucorrhea
Measles
Menstruation
MORNING SICKNESS
MOUTH SORES
NAUSEA

Nervousness
PREGNANCY
Stomach
Teething
Throat, sore
Urinary problems
Uterus, prolapsed
VOMITING

REDMOND CLAY   (red-mūnd klā)
(Montmorillonite)
Parts used: Clay

Redmond Clay is used externally for skin problems. It is good to have around for stings or bug bites. It is useful for expelling worms from the intestinal tract, and for beauty marks, muscle sprains and wounds. It can also be used for fevers (forehead and back of neck). It will absorb poisons in the stomach quickly if taken with a glass of water.

Acne
BEE STINGS
Bug bites

Poisoning, internal
SKIN PROBLEMS
Worms

RHUBARB   (rōō'-bārb')
(Rheum palmatum)
Parts used: Root

Rhubarb is a mild stimulating tonic to the liver, gall ducts and mucous membranes in the intestines. It acts as a laxative, clearing the cause of intestinal irritants and checking diarrhea with its astringent action. Rhubarb cleanses the mucous membrane of viscid material. Rhubarb is useful when the stomach is weak and the bowels relaxed at the same time. It acts as a gentle cathartic. It has been used in almost all thyrhoid diseases when fecal matter is accumulated in the intestines or to prevent such an accumulation. It is very useful in toxic blood conditions from excessive intake of meat.

Rhubarb contains vitamins A, C and B-complex. It is high in calcium. It also contains sodium, potassium, some iron, sulphur, phosphorus, cobalt, nickel and tin.

Anemia	Dysentery
Colitis	Jaundice
COLON	Gallbladder
Constipation	Headaches
DIARRHEA	LIVER PROBLEMS
Digestion aids	Stomach

ROSE HIPS   (rōz hīps)
(Rosa species)
Parts used: Fruit

Rose Hips helps play an important role in treatment where vitamins A, E, and C and Rutin are needed. This herb is very nourishing to the skin. It contains natural fruit sugar. A Swiss herbalist, Father Kunzle, recommends the use of Rose Hips to help expel kidney stones. It helps prevent infections and also helps when infections develop.

Rose Hips is very high in vitamin B-complex and is very rich in vitamins A, E, C and Rutin. It also contains vitamins D, and P. It is high in organic iron and calcium. It has some sodium, potassium, sulphur, silica, and niacin.

Arteriosclerosis	Fever
Bites	FLU
BLOOD PURIFER	Headaches
Bruises	INFECTIONS
CANCER	Kidney stones
Circulation	Mouth sores
COLDS	NERVOUSNESS
Contagious diseases	Psoriasis
Cramps	Stings
Dizziness	Stress
Earaches	THROAT, SORE

ROSEMARY (rōz'-mārē)
(Rosmarinus officinalis)
Parts used: Leaves

Rosemary is a strong stimulant especially of the circulatory system and pelvic region. It is considered a proven heart tonic which is not a drastic drug. It is a treatment for high blood pressure. It is used externally for wounds of all kinds including bites and stings. It is excellent for all womens' ailments. It helps regulate menses, and should be thought of when there are pains from the uterus followed by hemorrhage. It is a good tonic for the reproductive organs. Rosemary tea will help relieve hysterical depression and is very good for headaches caused by nerves as it is stimulating to the nervous system. It has been considered to be one of the most powerful remedies to strengthen the nervous system. In colds or flu, Rosemary can be taken in the early stages as a warm infusion, and may be used as a cooling tea when there is restlessness, nervousness, and insomnia. Rosemary, sage, and vervain in equal parts makes an antiseptic drink for fevers. It has been known for preventing premature baldness and being a stimulant for increased activity of the "hair-bulbs."

It contains vitamins A and C. It is high in calcium. It contains iron, magnesium, phosphorus, potassium, sodium and zinc.

BAD BREATH	HEART TONIC
Baldness	High blood pressure
Circulation	Hysteria
Convulsions	Liver
Digestion	Memory
Dropsy	Menstruation
Eczema	Nervousness
Eye wash	Prostate
Female problems	Spasms
Gall bladder	Sores, open
Gas	Stings, external
Hair (stimulates)	STOMACH DISORDER
HEADACHES, MIGRAINE	Wounds

RUE   (rōo)
(Ruta graveolens)
Parts used: The Herb

Rue has the ability to expel poisons from the system and has been used for snake bites, scorpion, spider or jellyfish bites. Rue has been found very effective in preserving the sight by strengthening the ocular muscles. Rue helps remove deposits that through age are liable to form in the tendons and joints especially the joints of the wrist. It should not be used by pregnant women. Because of its emetic properties, it should not be taken with meals.

Rue contains large amounts of rutin (vitamin P), which is known for its ability to strengthen capillaries and veins. The U.S. department of agriculture found that rutin was very effective in treating high blood pressure and also helps to harden the bones and teeth.

Arteriosclerosis
BLOOD PRESSURE, HIGH
Bruising, easy
Circulation, poor
Colic
Convulsions
Coughs
CRAMPS
Croup, spasmodic
Earaches
Eye ailments
Epilepsy
Female problems
HYPERTENSION
HYSTERIA
Insanity
Malaria
Metabolism (improves)
MUSCLES, STRAINED
NEURALGIA
NERVOUS DISORDER
Nosebleeds, chronic
Poisons (antidote for)
SCIATICA
TENDONS, STRAINED
TRAUMA
Typhoid
VARICOSE VEINS
Whooping cough
Worms

SAFFLOWER (saf'-lau-er)
(Carthamus tinctorius)
Parts used: Flowers

Safflower has become a popular remedy for jaundice, sluggish liver and gallbladder problems. It is also used for children's complaints in eruptive diseases and fevers.

It has the ability to remove hard phlegm from the system. It clears the lungs and helps in pulmonary tuberculosis.

Safflower has gained popularity the past few years because of the fixed oil in the seeds and their kernel. It is supposed to help with the cholesterol level in the blood.

It contains vitamin K.

Boils, external	Measles
Chickenpox	Menstruation
DELIRIUM	Mumps
DIGESTION	PHLEGM
FEVERS	Poison ivy
Gallbladder	Scarlet fever
GOUT	SWEATING
JAUNDICE	Tuberculosis
Heart (strengthens)	URIC ACID
Hysteria	URINARY PROBLEMS
LIVER	

SAFFRON (sāf'-ran)
(Crocus satirus)
Parts used: Flowers

Saffron soothes the membranes of the stomach and colon. It helps reduce cholesterol levels by neutralizing uric-acid build up in the system. It has been known to prevent heart disease. In Valencia, Spain, Saffron is eaten daily and little heart disease exists there.

Saffron contains vitamins A and B12. It contains potassium, some calcium, phosphorus, sodium, and lactic acid.

Arthritis	Jaundice
Bronchitis	MEASLES
Coughs	Menstruation
Digestion	Psoriasis
FEVERS	RHEUMATISM
Gas	SCARLET FEVER
GOUT	Skin diseases
Headaches	Stomach disorders
Heartburn	Tuberculosis
Hyperglycemia	Ulcers, internal
Hypoglycemia	Uterine hemorrhages
Insomnia	Water retention

SAGE   (sāj)
(Salvia officinalis)
Parts used: Leaves

Sage is used for excessive mucus discharges, nasal catarrh and indurated sores and excessive secretions of saliva.

This herb was used anciently as a staple remedy in the home and was thought to save and prolong life. The fresh leaves were used by chewing them for infections of the mouth and throat.

Sage is beneficial for mental exhaustion and strengthening the ability to concentrate. It improves the memory and has been used to cure some types of insanity.

It was used as a lotion to heal sores and other skin eruptions. It will stop bleeding from wounds.

Sage contains vitamins A and C, vitamin B-complex. It has a lot of calcium and potassium. It also contains sulphur, silicon, phosphorus, and sodium.

Brain, (stimulates)	Colds
Bladder infection	COUGHS
Blood infections	Diarrhea

DIGESTION
Dysentery
FEVERS
Flu
Gravel
GUMS, SORE
Hair growth
Headaches
Lactation (stops)
Laryngitis
Lung congestion
MEMORY (IMPROVES)
MOUTH SORES
NAUSEA

NERVES
Night sweats
Palsy
Parasites
Phlegm
Sinus congestion
Snake bites
Teeth cleanser
THROAT, SORE
Tonsillitis
Ulcers
Worms
Yeast infections

ST. JOHNSWORT (sānt jönz'-wert)
(Hypericum perforatum)
Parts used: The Herb

St. Johnswort is very helpful for obstructions of phlegm in the chest and lungs. It has been known in cases of bronchitis to eliminate all signs of the condition. It is excellent for internal bleeding. The seeds steeped in boiling water expel congealed blood from the stomach caused by bruises, falls, or bursting veins. It is useful in healing wounds, and excellent for dirty, septic wounds and has been used in cases of putrid leg ulcers when nothing else would heal. It helps in depression and mild pain in the stomach, intestines and gall bladder. It is effective in headaches with excitability, hysteria, neuralgia, especially such symptoms occurring at the menopause, such as brain-lag, or heavy feeling in the head, or with throbbing on the top of the head. St. Johnswort is useful in swellings, neglected cuts, abscesses, boils and bad insect stings.

AFTERPAINS
Appetite
BED WETTING
Bites, insect

Bleeding (internal)
Blood purifier
Boils
BRONCHITIS

Breasts, caked
Diarrhea
Dysentery
Hemorrhaging
Hysteria
Insomnia
Jaundice
LUNG CONGESTION
Melancholy
Menopause
MENSTRUATION,
  PAINFUL
Nervousness
Skin problems
Spasms
Tumors
Ulcers
URINE, SUPPRESSED
UTERINE
Whitlows
Worms
Wounds

SARSAPARILLA (sās'-pa-rīl'-a)
(Smilax ornata)
Parts used: Root

Sarsaparilla is a valuable herb used in glandular balance formulas. Its stimulating properties are noted for increasing the metabolic rate.

It contains an important male hormone known as testosterone which is an important hair-growing hormone.

It also contains progesterone, another valuable hormone which is normally produced by the ovaries in the female.

It increases circulation to rheumatic joints. It stimulates breathing in problems of congestion.

Sarsaparilla contains vitamin B-complex, vitamins A, C and D. It also contains iron, manganese, sodium, silicon, sulphur, copper, zinc, and iodine.

Age spots
BLOOD PURIFIER
Catarrh
Colds
Dropsy
Eyes, sore
Fevers
GAS
Gout
JOINT ACHES
HORMONE HERB
Menopause

Physical debility
Psoriasis
Rheumatism, chronic
Ring worm
Sexual impotence
Scrofula

SKIN DISEASES
Skin parasites
Sores
Tetters
Veneral diseases

SASSAFRAS (sās'-a-frās')
(Sassafras officinale)
Parts used: Root Bark

Sassafras stimulates the action of the liver to clear toxins from the system, making a good tonic especially after childbirth. It has been used as a pain reliever and also to treat venereal diseases. The Indians used an infusion of Sassafras roots to bring down a fever. Sassafras and Burdock are excellent as an appetite-control hormone tonic. The ingredients of these herbs aid the pituitary gland in releasing an ample supply of protein, which helps adjust hormone balance in the body.

ACNE
Afterpains
Bladder problems
BLOOD PURIFIER
Boils
Bronchitis
Colic
Cramps, stomach
Diarrhea
Gas
Kidney problems

OBESITY
Perspiration, increases
Poison ivy and oak
PSORIASIS
Rheumatism
SKIN DISEASES
Spasms
Toothache
Varicose ulcers
WATER RETENTION

SAW PALMETTO (sō pal-met'-ō)
(Serenoa serrulata)
Parts used: Fruit

Saw Palmetto is recommended in all wasting diseases because it has an effect upon all the glandular tissues. It is also useful on all diseases of the reproductive glands.

The crushed root was used by the Indians for sore breasts. It has been said to increase the size of small breasts.

It is used for mucous membranes of the throat, nose and all air passages, chronic bronchitis and lung asthma.

Saw Palmetto contains vitamin A.

Asthma	Lung congestion
Bladder diseases	Mucous (excess)
BREASTS	Nerves
Bronchitis, chronic	Neuralgia
Catarrhal problems	REPRODUCTIVE ORGANS
Colds, head	SEX STIMULANT
Diabetes	Tonic
DIGESTION	Urinary problems
GLANDS	WEIGHT (INCREASES)
Kidney diseases	

SCHIZANDRA   (sch' zăn-drå)
(Schisandra chinensis)
Part used: The berries

Schizandra is an herb capable of increasing the body's immune system and protecting the body against stress. It contains properties to increase energy, nourish the veins and improve vision.

It is an adaptogen herb that increases the energy supply of cells in the brain, muscles, liver, kidney, glands, nerves and in the entire body. It protects against free radical damage. It helps to balance body functions, normalizes body systems and speeds recovery after surgery. It can protect against radiation, counteracts the effects of sugar, boosts stamina, normalizes blood sugar and blood pressure and also protects against infections. It also protects the body when under undue stress.

Schizandra is high in vitamin C, magnesium, phosphorus, and also contains iron, potassium, calcium, manganese, selenium, silicon and sodium.

Aging
Atherosclerosis
Blood pressure, normalizes
Coughs
Digestive problems
ENERGY, INCREASES
Fatigue
Gastritis, chronic
Hepatitis
Infections
Insomnia

Kidney problems
Lung problems
MENTAL ALERTNESS
Motion Sickness
NERVOUS DISORDER
Radiation
STRESS
Tonic
Uterine problems
Vision, improves

SCULLCAP   (skūl-kāp)
(Scutellaria lateriflora)
Parts used: The Herb

Scullcap is said to be stimulating to the nerves as quinine without harmful side-effects. It is called a food for the nerves, supporting and strengthening them as it gives immediate relief of all chronic and acute diseases stemming from nervous affections and debility.

Scullcap is said to be one of the herbs used traditionally to cure infertility. It is also said to regulate undue sexual desires. Scullcap mixed with Pennyroyal has been used successfully as a female remedy for cramps and severe pain caused by suppressed menstruation due to colds.

Scullcap is high in calcium, potassium, and magnesium. It also contains vitamins C, E, iron and zinc.

Aches
Alcoholism
Blood pressure

Childhood diseases
CONVULSIONS
Delirium

Drug withdrawal
EPILEPSY
FEVERS (REDUCES)
Fits
Hangover
Headaches
HIGH BLOOD PRESSURE
Hydrophobia
Hypertension
Hysteria
Hypoglycemia
INFERTILITY
Insanity
INSOMNIA
Lock-jaw
NERVES

Neuralgia
Pain
Palsy
Parkinson's diseases
Poisonous bites
Rabies
RESTLESSNESS
Rheumatism
Rickets
Spasms
Spinal meningitis
St. Vitus dance
Thyroid problems
Tremors
Urinary

SENEGA   (se'-nē-gà)
(Polygala senega)
Parts used: Root

Senega is used as an expectorant in respiratory problems. In normal doses it stimulates the secretions, acting particularly as an expectorant. It has been said to be an excellent antidote for many poisons. It is useful in the second stage of acute bronchial catarrh or pneumonia. It increases the secretions and circulation and is useful when there is prostration from blood poisoning, small pox, asthma, and diseases of the lungs.

Senega contains magnesium, iron, tin, lead and aluminum in small amounts.

ASTHMA
Blood poisoning
BRONCHITIS, CHRONIC
CATARRH, CHRONIC
CROUP
Dropsy
Drugs, (side effects)
LUNG CONGESTION

MUCUS (IN TISSUES)
Pleurisy
PNEUMONIA
Rheumatism
Small pox
SNAKEBITES
Whooping cough

SENNA   (sén-a)
(Cassia acutifolia)
Parts used: Leaves and Pods

Senna is a very useful laxative because it increases the intestinal peristaltic movements. It has a strong laxative effect on the entire intestinal tract, especially the colon and large intestines. It should always be taken with carminative herbs such as ginger or fennel to prevent bowel cramps. It should not be used in cases of inflammation of the stomach.

It is a very useful herb to cleanse the system during fasting and in all fevers. Used as a laxative, it tones and restores the digestive system as it thoroughly cleans it.

Bad breath	Menstruation
Biliousness	Obesity
Colic	Pimples
CONSTIPATION	Rheumatism
Gallstones	Skin diseases
Gout	Sores, mouth
JAUNDICE	WORMS

SHEPHERD'S PURSE   (shép-herdz pers)
(Capsella bursa-pastoris)
Parts used: The Whole Plant

Shepherd's Purse is used for cases of hemorrhages after childbirth, excessive menstruation and for internal bleeding of the lungs, colon and hemorrhoids. It helps to constrict the blood vessels and is therefore used to regulate blood pressure and heart action whether there is high or low pressure.

It acts as a stimulant and moderate tonic for catarrh of the urinary tract indicated by mucus in the urine.

Shepherd's Purse is high in vitamin C. It also contains vitamins E and K. It has iron, magnesium, calcium, potassium, tin, zinc, sodium, and sulphur.

Arteriosclerosis
BLEEDING
BLOOD PRESSURE
BLOODY URINE
Bowels
Constipation
Diarrhea
Dropsy
Dysentery
EAR AILMENTS

Heart
Hemorrhage
Kidney problems
Lumbago
MENSTRUATION,
  PAINFUL
Uterus
Vagina
Water retention

SLIPPERY ELM   (slip'-e-re elm)
(Ulmus fulva)
Parts used: Inner Bark

Slippery Elm has the ability to neutralize stomach acidity and to absorb foul gases. It aids in the digestion of milk. It acts as a buffer against irritations and inflammations of the mucous membranes.

Slippery Elm's properties help assist the activity of the adrenal glands. It helps to boost the output of the cortin hormone, which helps send a stream of blood-building substances through the system.

It is used as a food whenever there is difficulty holding and digesting food.

It draws out impurities and heals all parts of the body. It is an excellent remedy for the respiratory system. It has the ability to remove mucus with stronger force than other herbs.

Slippery Elm contains vitamins E, F, K and P. It also contains iron, sodium, calcium, selenium, iodine, copper, zinc and some potassium and phosphorus.

Appendicitis
ASTHMA
Bladder problems
Boils
Bowels
BRONCHITIS

BURNS
Cancer
COLITIS
COLON
COUGHS
Constipation

Croup
DIAPER RASH
DIARRHEA
DIGESTION
Diphtheria
Dysentery
Female problems
Hemorrhoids
Herpes
Inflammations
Laxative
LUNG PROBLEMS
Pain
Phlegm

Plague, white
Pneumonia
Poison ivy, external
Sores
Syphilis
Throat, sore
Tuberculosis
Tumors
Ulcers
Urinary problems
Vaginal irritations
Worms
Wounds
Whooping cough

SPEARMINT (spier-ment)
(Mentha viridis)
Parts used: Leaves

Spearmint is a valuable herb for even the sickest person to tolerate because there is no toxicity. It is excellent in stopping vomiting in pregnancy. The oil in the leaves works on the salivary glands to aid in digestion. It stimulates gastric secretion and is credited with an action of biliary secretion.

It is gentle and effective for colic in babies.

Spearmint is an excellent source of vitamins C and A. It contains B-complex, calcium, sulphur, iron, iodine, magnesium and potassium.

Bladder inflammation
Chills
COLDS
COLIC
Cramps
Dizziness
Dropsy
Fever
FLU

GAS
Hysteria
Indigestion
Kidney inflammation
NAUSEA
Spasms
Stones
Urine, suppressed
VOMITING

SPIKENARD   (spīk'-nard)
(Aralia racemosa)
Parts used: Root

Spikenard as a tea has been used before labor to make childbirth easier and to help shorten the ordeal. It is useful for uric acid buildup in the system and also in rheumatic disorders. Spikenard has been combined with other herbs to purify as well as build the blood. It is slightly expectorant in its effect and is useful in cough syrups along with other herbs. The properties of the plant are very close to Ginseng. The Russians use the roots as a general tonic and stimulant, especially for physical and mental exhaustion.

ASTHMA	Hemorrhoids
Backache	Inflammation
Blood purifier	Leucorrhea
Chest pains	Lung congestion
CHILD BIRTH	Prolapsus ani
COUGH	RHEUMATISM
Diarrhea	Skin problems
Hay fever	Venereal diseases

SPIRULINA   (spir-ŭ-li' nå)
(spirulina pratensis)
Part used: Whole herb

Spirulina is used in weight control diets. It provides nutrients that satisfy the hidden hunger the body craves when it is not getting enough essential nutrition. It is an easily digestible food to strengthen the body and provide nutrients when the body is weak, either after an acute disease or during a chronic disease. It will help build vitality the body needs. It will purify and build the blood to nourish all the cells.

Spirulina is a natural food supplement to help balance the diet. It is considered one of Nature's whole foods. It is easy to digest and assimilate.

Spirulina is rich in protein, chlorophyll and essential fatty acids. It is high in vitamin A and B vitamins, including B_{12}. It is high in iron, magnesium and phosphorus. It contains calcium, potassium, sodium, vitamin C and E. It contains about all the nutrients required by the body.

Anemia
Appetite suppressant
BLOOD BUILDER
Blood pressure, regulates
CHRONIC DISEASES
Diets

FOOD SUPPLEMENT
Goiter
Gout
Hypoglycemia
Skin problems
TONIC

STEVIA (ste-veå)
(Stevia rebaudiana)
Parts Used: Leaves

Stevia is a natural sweetener, 30 to 100 times sweeter than sugar. Small amounts go a long way and there is no after taste like sugar substitutes. Stevia is used in Paraguay and Brazil and has been cultivated and used as a natural sweetener for centuries.

Research is Japan found Stevia to be nontoxic and safe to use. They use it in soy sauce, chewing gum and mouthwash. It is a non-fattening sweetener and can be used in cold and hot cereals and in herbal teas.

Stevia is high in chromium, (helps to establish blood sugar), manganese, potassium, selenium, silicon, sodium and vitamin A. Also contains iron, niacin, phosphorus, riboflavin, thiamine, vitamin C, and zinc.

Addictions   OBESITY
DIABETES   TOBACCO CRAVINGS
FOOD CRAVINGS   SUGAR SUBSTITUTE
Hypertension
Hypoglycemia

SQUAWVINE   (skwŏ'-vīn)
(Mitchella repens)
Parts used: The Herb

Squawvine is especially helpful in childbirth. It strengthens the uterus for safe and effective childbirth. It is called a uterine tonic because it relieves congestion of the uterus and ovaries. It helps restore the menstrual function. It contains antiseptic properties, which is ideal for any kind of vaginal infection. It is also beneficial as a natural sedative on the nerves. It is best used with other herbs such as Red Raspberry.

Bites, snake   Leucorrhea
CHILDBIRTH, EASIER   MENSTRUATION
Diarrhea   Nerves
Dropsy   SKIN PROBLEMS
EYE, SORE   Syphilis
Female problems   UTERINE DISORDERS
Gonorrhea   Urinary problems
Gravel   Varicose veins
Hemorrhoids   Water retention
Insomnia   Wounds
LACTATION

STILLINGIA   (stil-in'-gia)
(Stillingia ligustina)
Parts used: Root

Stillingia is an effective glandular stimulant, as well as an activator for the liver. It is said to be valuable to rid the system of toxic drugs when using chemotherapy treatment for cancer. It is one of the most powerful herb alteratives known. It should be used with caution and is used best in combination with other herbs to complement its effectiveness. It is especially useful when a stimulant is needed for the liver.

ACNE	RESPIRATORY
BLOOD PURIFIER	PROBLEMS
Bronchitis	SKIN PROBLEMS
Constipation	SYPHILIS
ECZEMA	Throat, sore
LIVER PROBLEMS	Urinary problems

STRAWBERRY   (strô'-bé-rē)
(Fragaria vesca)
Parts used: Leaves

Strawberry tones the appetitie and aids in the overall conditions of the system. It acts as a cleanser for the stomach and is useful for bowel troubles. It is a safe and useful herb for children.

It has been used for eczema, externally and internally. Discolored teeth or teeth encrusted with tarter can be cleaned with strawberry juice.

The roots are especially useful for obstinate dysentery.

Strawberry leaves are rich in iron. They contain vitamins A and C. Strawberry leaves also contain some B-complex, calcium, phosphorus, and potassium.

Acne
BLOOD PURIFIER
Bowel problems
DIARRHEA
Dysentery
ECZEMA
Fevers
High blood pressure, lowers
INTESTINES

Jaundice
Lactation
MISCARRIAGE
 (PREVENTS)
Nerves
NIGHT SWEATS
STOMACH, CLEANS
URINARY PROBLEMS
Vomiting

SUMA   (su'ma)
(Pfaffia paniculata)
Parts used: Bark and the Root

Suma is an adaptogen herb, one to heal and prevent disease. It relieves stress and helps the body to adapt to many and varied environment and psychological stresses. It is an herb that benefits both men and women, to restore sexual function, protect against viral infections and benefits in cancer.

Research in Japan discovered a unique chemical in Suma that tends to inhibit tumor cell growth. It is another nutrient to help protect the immune system. It contains allantoin (also found in comfrey), known to promote the healing of wounds and new cell growth.

It contains two plant hormones, sitosterol and stipmasterol, found beneficial to human metabolism, by increasing heart circulation and decreasing high blood cholesterol levels in the blood. Sitosterol enhances the body's natural production of estrogen when the body is depleted. It prevents the random release of free radicals. The Portuguese call it "Para Todo", which means "for everything."

Suma contains germanium, iron and magnesium.

Anemia
Arthritis

Balance hormones
Bronchitis

Cancer
CIRCULATION PROBLEMS
CHOLESTEROL
CHRONIC DISEASES
Colds
Diabetes
Emotional swings
Energy booster
FATIGUE
Heart disease
HORMONE REGULATOR
Hot flashes
Hypoglycemia

IMMUNE SYSTEM
Joint diseases
Menopause systems
Premenstrual problems
Osteomelitis
Osteoporosis
Skin problems
STRESS
Strokes
TONIC
Tumors
Wounds

TAHEEBO   (te-hē′-bō)
(Tabebuia avellanedae)
Parts used: Inner Bark

This herb also goes by the name of Pau D' Arco, or Ipe Roxo. The herb is found in South America. It is used in some hospitals in South America with great success on Cancer patients. It is a powerful antibiotic with virus-killing properties. Taheebo is said to contain compounds which seem to attack the cause of disease. It is said that one of its main action is that it puts the body into a defensive posture, to give it the energy needed to defend itself and to help resist diseases.

Taheebo contains a high amount of iron, which aids in the proper assimilation of nutrients, and the elimination of wastes.

Anemia
Arteriosclerosis

Asthma
BLOOD BUILDER

Bronchitis
CANCER, ALL TYPES
Colitis
Cystitis
Diabetes
Eczema
Eyelids (paralysis)
Fistulas
Gastritis
Gonorrhea
Hemorrhages
Hernias
Hodgkins Disease
Infections
LEUKEMIA
Liver ailments
Lupus

Nephritis
Osteomyelitis
Parkinson's Disease
PAIN (RELIEVES)
Polyps
Prostatitis
Psoriasis
Rheumatism
Ringworm
SKIN CANCER
Skin sores
Spleen infections
Syphilis
TONIC
Ulcers
Varicose ulcers
Wounds

THYME   (tīm)
(Thymus vulgaris)
Parts used: The Herb

Thyme is a powerful antiseptic and a general tonic with healing powers. It is said to be used in cases of anemia, bronchial, and intestinal disturbances. It is used as an antiseptic against tooth decay. It destroys fungal infections as in athlete's foot and skin parasites such as crabs and lice.

Culpeper says it kills worms in the belly, and that an ointment of Thyme takes away any hot swelling and warts.

Thyme contains B-complex, vitamins C and D. It also contains a lot of iodine, some sodium, silicon and sulphur.

Appetite stimulant
Asthma
Bowel problems
BRONCHITIS, ACUTE
Bruises
Catarrh
COLIC

Diarrhea
DIGESTION
Epilepsy
Fainting
Fevers
GAS
Gastritis

GOUT, EXTERNAL
HEADACHES
Heartburn
Hysteria
Infection, internal
LARYNGITIS
Leprosy
LUNG CONGESTION
Mastitis
Menstruation, suppressed
Nightmares
Paralysis

Parasites
Perspiration (promotes)
Rheumatism
SCIATICA
Sinus problems
Sprains
Stomach problems
THROAT PROBLEMS
Uterine problems
Warts
WHOOPING COUGH
WORMS

UVA URSI   (yū-va yur'-si)
(Arctostaphylos uva-ursi) (Bearberry)
Parts used: Leaves

Uva Ursi strengthens and tones the urinary passages. It is especially beneficial for bladder and kidney infections. It increases the flow of urine. It is useful in inflammatory diseases of the urinary tract, arthritis, and cystitis. This herb is best known as the diabetes remedy for excessive sugar. It should not be used during pregnancy in any large quantities because of the possibility of decreased circulation to the fetus. Tincture of Uva Ursi was routinely prescribed in many European hospitals as a post partum medicine to reduce hemorrhaging and help restore the womb to normal size.

Arthritis
Bedwetting
BLADDER INFECTIONS
Bronchitis
BRIGHT'S DISEASE
CYSTITIS
DIABETES
Diarrhea
Dysentery
Female troubles
Gallstones

GONORRHEA
Gravel
Hemorrhoids
KIDNEY INFECTIONS
Liver
Lung congestion
Menstruation, excessive
NEPHRITIS
Pancreas
Piles
Prostate weakness

SPLEEN   URETHRITIS, CHRONIC
Uric acid, excess   UTERINE, ULCERATION

VALERIAN   (veli̇r'-ien)
(Valeriana officinalis)
Parts used: Root

Valerian is a strong nervine and is very helpful for insomniacs. It contains an essential oil and alkaloids which combine to produce a calming sedative effect. It can be used as a tranquilizer but leaves one feeling refreshed rather than sluggish. It is known as a safe non-narcotic herbal sedative and has been recommended in anxiety states.

Valerian is commonly used with other herbs for nervous tension. It is also useful in pain-relieving remedies and for its relaxing properties for muscle spasms.

Valerian is usually recommended for short-term use. Prolonged or excessive use can cause mental depression in some people. It is usually not recommended for small children.

Valerian is rich in magnesium, potassium, copper, some lead and zinc.

Alcoholism   Insomnia
Bronchial spasms   Measles
Colds   Menstruation (promotes)
Coughs   Muscle pain
CONVULSIONS   NERVOUSNESS
Despondency   PAIN
Drug addiction   Palpitations
Epilepsy   Palsy
Gravel bladder   Scarlet fever
Head, congestion   Shock
HIGH BLOOD PRESSURE   Spasms
HYSTERIA   Ulcers
HYPOCHONDRIA   Worms (expels)

VIOLET   (vī'-ō-let)
(Viola odorata)
Parts used: Flowers and Leaves

Violet is very effective in healing internal ulcers. It is used internally and externally for tumors, boils, abscesses, pimples, swollen glands and malignant growths. The properties in violet leaves and flowers seem to have abilities to reach places only the blood and lymphatic fluids penetrate.

It is useful in difficult breathing when the causes are from morbid accumulations of material in the stomach and bowels causing gas, distention and pressure.

Violet contains vitamins A and C.

ASTHMA	Scrofula
Breathing, difficult	SINUS CATARRH
BRONCHITIS	Sores
CANCER	Syphilis
COLDS, HEAD CONGES-TION	Throat, sore
COUGHS	TUMORS
Gout	ULCERS
Headaches	Whooping cough

WATERCRESS   (wät'-er kres)
(Nasturtium officinale)
Parts used: The Whole Plant

Watercress is used principally as a tonic, for regulating the metabolism and the flow of bile. It helps in increasing physical endurance and stamina.

Watercress eaten fresh daily is a very useful blood purifier and tonic to help supply needed vitamins and minerals. The juice of the leaves have been applied to the face for freckles, pimples, spots and left overnight then washed off in the morning.

Used as a cough medicine, Watercress soaked in honey has been found beneficial. Watercress is an overall excellent food for enriching the blood in anemia and a good remedy in most blood and skin disorders.

Experiments have proven that the dried leaves contain three times as much vitamin C as the leaves of lettuce.

Watercress is very rich in vitamins A, C, and D. It is one of the best sources of vitamin E. It also contains vitamins B and G. It is high in iron, iodine, calcium, copper, sulphur and manganese.

Acne	Lactation
ANEMIA	LIVER PROBLEMS
Appetite (increases)	Mental disorders
CRAMPS	NERVOUS AILMENTS
Cysts	RHEUMATISM
Eczema	TONIC
Heart (strengthens)	Tuberculosis
Joints, stiff	Tumors, internal
KIDNEY PROBLEMS	Uterine cysts
Kidney stones	WATER RETENTION

WHITE OAK BARK   (wĭt-ōk bärk)
(Quercus alba)
Parts used: Bark

White Oak Bark contains strong astringent properties that can be used for both external and internal bleeding. It is an excellent cleanser for inflamed areas of the skin and mucous membranes. It heals damaged tissues in the stomach and intestines. It has been used for excess stomach mucus which causes common complaint of sinus congestion and post-nasal drip.

It relieves the stomach by strengthening it for better internal absorption and secretion and thus improving metabolism.

A tea of the bark can be used with success as a wash for gum infection, gargle for sore throats, and as an intestinal tonic for diarrhea. It is also used as an antidote for drug allergies and chemotherapy side-effects.

It is useful for inflammations, abrasions, and cuts. It has a clotting, shrinking and antiseptic effect.

It contains vitamin B12, calcium, phosphorus, potassium and iodine. It also contains sulphur, iron, sodium, cobalt, lead, strontium, and tin.

Bites, insect and snake
Bladder problems
BLEEDING, INTERNAL AND EXTERNAL
BLOODY URINE
Cancer, prostate
Dental problems
Diarrhea
Fever (reduces)
Gangrene
Glandular swellings
Goiter
Gums, sore
HEMORRHOIDS
Indigestion
Kidneys
Liver
MENSTRUAL PROBLEMS
MOUTH SORES
Nausea
Pyorrhea
SKIN IRRITATIONS
Spleen problems
TEETH
THROAT, STREP
Tonsillitis
ULCERS
Uterus
Vagina
VARICOSE VEINS
Venereal diseases
Vomiting
WORMS, PIN
Wounds, external

WHITE PINE BARK   (wīt pīn bärk)
(Pinus strobus)
Parts used: Bark

White Pine Bark is said to be an excellent expectorant, to reduce mucus secretions in common colds and helps in its elimination. The bark contains medicinal properties as well as food value.

The Indians soaked the bark in water until it became soft and then applied it to wounds. They also boiled the inner bark of saplings and drank the liquid for dysentery.

White pine bark is rich in vitamin C and has some vitamin A. It contains iodine, calcium, copper, sodium, nickel, zinc and manganese.

BRONCHITIS	Lung congestion
CATARRH	MUCUS
Colds	Rheumatism
Croup	Scurvy
DYSENTERY	Strep throat
Flu	Tonsillitis
Kidney problems	Whooping cough
LARYNGITIS	

WILD CHERRY   (wīld cher'ē)
(Prunus virginiana)
Parts used: Bark

Wild Cherry is considered a very useful expectorant. It is a valuable remedy for all catarrhal conditions.

It contains a volatile oil which acts as a local stimulant in the alimentary canal which helps aid in digestion. It is a useful tonic for those convalescing. It tones up the entire system.

It is also beneficial for bronchial disorders caused by the hardened accumulation of mucus.

ASTHMA	Heart palpitation
BRONCHITIS	HIGH BLOOD PRESSURE
CATARRH	MUCUS, HARDENED
COUGHS (LOOSENS)	PHLEGM (LOOSENS)
Diarrhea	Scrofula
Dyspepsia	Spasms
Eye sight	Stomach, irritated
FEVER, HECTIC	TUBERCULOSIS
Flu	Worms, intestinal
Gall bladder	

WILD LETTUCE   (wīld let'-es)
(Lactuca virosa)
Parts used: The Whole Plant

Wild Lettuce has been used to increase urine flow and to soothe sore and chapped skin. The Indians used it as a tea for lactation.

The leaves contain sedative properties that act somewhat like morphine, only milder. It is the dried leaves which are used to induce sleep and treat severe nervous disorders.

The Indians also used the juice of the plant to relieve poison ivy.

Asthma
BRONCHITIS
Colic
Coughs
CRAMPS
Diarrhea
Dropsy

Insomnia
Lactation
NERVOUS DISORDERS
PAIN, CHRONIC
Spasms
WHOOPING COUGH

WILD YAM   (wīld yam)
(Dioscorea villosa)
Parts used: Root

Wild Yam is useful in glandular balance formulas for treating nausea in pregnant women. It is said to be an excellent preventative of miscarriage and also useful for cramps in the region of the uterus during the later stages of pregnancy.

It is useful for pain with gallstones and it will relax the muscular fiber and soothe the nerves.

ARTHRITIS
ASTHMA, SPASMODIC
Boils
BOWEL SPASMS
Bronchitis

Catarrh, stomach
Cholera
COLIC, BILIOUS
GAS
Hiccough, spasmodic

Jaundice
LIVER PROBLEMS
MENSTRUAL CRAMPS
MUSCLE PAIN
NAUSEA (FROM
  PREGNANCY)

Nervousness
Neuralgia
Rheumatism
Scabies
Whooping cough

WILLOW (wil-ō)
(Salix)
Parts used: Bark

Willow is valued as a nerve sedative because it leaves no depressing after-effects. It works like aspirin, except that it is mild on the stomach and is natural.

The bitter drink was made by steeping Willow bark and twigs in water for fever and chills and as a substitute for clinchona bark.

The Willow bark extract is helpful in cleansing and healing eyes that are inflamed or infected.

It has been called one of the essential first aid plants for the hiker. It has strong but benign antiseptic abilities for infected wounds, ulcerations, or eczema.

Bleeding
Chills
Corns
Dandruff
Diarrhea
Dysentery
Earache
ECZEMA
FEVER
Flu
Gout
Hay fever
HEADACHE
Heartburn
Impotence

Infection
Inflammation
Muscle, sore
NERVOUSNESS
Neuralgia
Night sweats
Ovarian pain
PAIN
RHEUMATISM
SEX DEPRESSANT
Tonsillitis
ULCERATION
Worms
WOUNDS

WINTERGREEN (wint-er-grēn)
(Gaultheria procumbens)
Parts used: Leaves, Oil

Wintergreen is very valuable when used in small doses. It stimulates the stomach, heart and respiration. It has a penetrating effect on every cell. It acts on the cause of pain.

As a tea or hot compress for headache, rheumatic pains, sciatica, or pains in the joints or muscles, it is beneficial.

An infusion may also be used as a gargle for sore throat or as a douche for leucorrhea.

Externally, the oil of Wintergreen has been used for rheumatism, warts, corns, callouses, cysts, and even tatoo marks.

ACHES	Leucorrhea
Cystitis	LUMBAGO
Diabetes	PAIN
Diphtheria	Rheumatic fever
Gas	Sciatica
GOUT	Throat gargle
HEADACHES, MIGRAINE	Urinary
Inflammation	Yeast infection

WITCH HAZEL (wich hā'-zel)
(Hamamelis virginiana)
Parts used: Bark

Witch Hazel is used externally as an alcohol extract for insect bites, varicose veins, burns, hemorrhoids and to stop bleeding wounds. It is used internally to help stop bleeding from the lungs, uterus and other internal organs. It is used as a mouth wash for bleeding gums and inflamed conditions of the mouth and throat. It is said to be harmless and safe to use and mild and gentle in action.

Witch Hazel contains vitamins C, E, K, and P. It also contains iodine, manganese, zinc, copper and selenium.

BLEEDING, INTERNAL	Muscles, sore
Bruises	Nervousness
Burns	Poison ivy
Cuts	Scalds
Diarrhea	Sinus
Dysentery	Sores
Eyes (bags)	Stings
GUMS	Swellings
Hemorrhage	Tuberculosis
HEMORRHOIDS	Tumors
Insect bites	VARICOSE VEINS
Menstruation, excess	Venereal disease
MUCOUS MEMBRANES	Wounds

WOOD BETONY   (wŭd bet'-ene)
(Betonica officinalis)
Parts used: The Herb

Wood Betony is an effective sedative for children and tranquilizer for adults. It is useful for head and facial pain. It works in cleansing impurities from the blood. It opens congested areas of the liver and spleen. It is said to be effective for many diseases. It preserves the liver and helps avoid the dangers of epidemic diseases.

Wood Betony contains magnesium, manganese and phosphorus.

Asthma, bronchial	FEVERS
Bladder	Gout
Bleeding, internal	HEADACHES, MIGRAINE
Blood, improves	Heartburn
Convulsions	Heart stimulant
DELIRIUM	HYSTERIA
Diarrhea	Indigestion
Epilepsy	Insanity
Fainting	JAUNDICE

Kidney
LIVER PROBLEMS
Lung congestion
NERVOUSNESS
Neuralgia
Night sweats
Pain

Palsy
Parasites
Perspiration
Stomach cramps
Varicose veins
WORMS

WORMWOOD (werm-wŭd)
(Artemisia absinthium)
Parts used: The Herb, Leaves

Wormwood has been useful for all complaints of the digestive system such as constipation and indigestion. It is useful to stimulate sweating in dry fevers and for stomach acidity. It is effective in promoting menstruation and has a stimulating effect on uterine circulation and will also help with cramps. It is best used in small quantities and for short periods of time. It is rarely given to children. It has been used externally and internally to check falling of hair and baldness.

Wormwood contains vitamin B-complex and vitamin C. It also contains manganese, calcium, potassium, sodium and small amounts of cobalt and tin.

Appetite, increase
Blood circulation
CONSTIPATION
CRAMPS, MENSTRUAL
DEBILITY
DIGESTION AIDS
Dropsy
Earaches
FEVER
Female problems
Gall bladder
Gout
Insect (repels)
JAUNDICE

Kidney problems
Labor pains (relieves)
LIVER PROBLEMS
MENSTRUATION
 (PROMOTES)
Morning sickness
Nausea
Obesity
Poisons (expels)
Rheumatism
STOMACH PROBLEMS
Tonic
WORMS

YARROW (yar-ō)
(Achillea millefolium)
Parts used: Flower

Yarrow is used as a tonic in helping to regulate the function of the liver. It tones the mucous membrane of the stomach and bowels and heals the glandular system. It acts as a blood cleanser and at the same time opening the pores to permit free perspiration for elimination of waste and relieving the kidneys.

The leaves are an effective first aid to stimulate clotting in cuts and abrasions.

It is one of the most valuable herbs having a wide range of uses. Yarrow has recently been mentioned as having properties as an anti-cancer agent.

Yarrow contains Vitamins A, C, E, and F and some Vitamin K. It contains manganese, copper, potassium, iodine and iron.

	Headaches
Abrasions	Hysteria
Ague	Jaundice
Appetite (stimulates)	LUNGS, HEMORRHAGE
Bladder	Malaria
BLOOD CLEANSER	MEASLES
BOWELS, HEMORRHAGE	Menstrual bleeding
Brights Disease	Nipples, sore
Bronchitis	NOSE BLEEDS
Bruises	Piles
Burns	PERSPIRATION,
Cancer	OBSTRUCTED
CATARRH	Pleurisy
Chicken Pox	Pneumonia
COLDS	Rheumatism
Cramps	Smallpox
Cuts	Stomach problems
Diarrhea (infants)	Sweating (promotes)
Epilepsy	Throat, inflamed
FEVERS	Typhoid Fever
FLU	Ulcers
Hair, falling out	Urine retention

YELLOW DOCK (yel'-ō dòk)
(Rumex crispus)
Parts used: Root

Yellow Dock is an astringent and blood purifier and is useful in treating diseases of the blood and chronic skin ailments. It is one of the best blood builders in the herb kingdom. It stimulates elimination, improving flow of bile and acting as a laxative.

It is a nutritive tonic very high in iron so it is very useful in treating anemia. It nourishes the spleen and liver and is therefore effective in treating jaundice, lymphatic problems, and skin eruptions.

Yellow Dock is rich in easily digestible plant iron. It is rich in vitamins A, and C, manganese and nickel.

ANEMIA
Bladder
Blood disorders
BLOOD PURIFIER
Bowels, bleeding
Bronchitis, chronic
Cancer
Constipation
Dyspepsia
Ears, running
ITCHING
EYELIDS, ULCERATED
Female weakness
Jaundice

Leprosy
Leukemia
LIVER CONGESTION
Lungs, bleeding
Lymphatic problems
RHEUMATISM
Scurvy
SKIN PROBLEMS
Spleen
Stomach problems
Thyroid glands
Tumors
Ulcers

YERBA SANTA (yer-be sàn'-tà)
(Eriodictyon californicum, Benth.)
Parts used: Leaves

Yerba Santa is a mild but useful decongestant. It is used for all forms of bronchial congestion. It is excellent in the remedy of chest conditions, acute and chronic. It is an herb that purifies the blood. Yerba Santa stimulates the salivary and other digestive secretions.

The Indians used the fresh or dried leaves as a poultice for broken and unbroken skin. It is used for pain in rheumatism, tired limbs and of swellings and sores.

ASTHMA	Flu
Bladder catarrh	Hemorrhoids
BRONCHIAL	HAY FEVER
CONGESTION	Kidney problems
Catarrh	Laryngitis, chronic
COLDS	Nose discharge
Coughs	Rheumatism
Diarrhea	Stomach aches
Dysentery	Throat, sore
Fever	Vomiting

YUCCA   (yúk-e)
(Yucca glauca)
Parts used: Root

Yucca was used by the Indians of the Southwest for skin disorders, eruptions, and slow-healing ulcerations. It was also used on cuts to stop bleeding and helps avoid inflammation. They also used the roots as a poultice on breaks and sprains and for rheumatism.

The properties of Yucca which help in arthritis and rheumatism are due to the plants' high content of steroid saponins, which are precursors to cortisone.

Some feel that the Yucca saponins improve the body's ability to produce its own cortisone by supplying materials needed to be manufactured in the adrenal glands.

The root contains a high content of vitamins A, B-complex, and some vitamin C. It is high in calcium, potassium, phosphorus, iron, manganese and copper.

Addison's Disease
ARTHRITIS
Blood purifier
Bursitis
Cholesterol, reduces
Dandruff
Gall Bladder
Gonorrhea
Inflammation, internal
Liver problems
RHEUMATISM
Skin irritations
Skin problems
Venereal disease

Natural Harmony of Combined Herbs

Combined herbs will have more than one function, consisting as it does of several substances which work together in natural harmony, and when taken over a period of time, combined herbs will condition reflexes in the body which will produce effects comparable to those of specific drugs, without being as drastic or producing unknown side-effects.

This works because the herbs trigger off neuro-chemical reflexes which in time become automatic and continue even after the person has stopped taking the herbs. The advantage with herbal combinations is that the body brings about its own recovery and is unlikely to be susceptible to the same complaint during or after convalescence.

Unlike orthodox drugs, which treat the symptoms, herbal combinations go right to the root of the disease and treat its cause.

The following herbal combinations have been used with great success by people all over the world.

I have heard stories from hundreds of people who have benefitted from using the following combinations.

Herb Combinations

The following combinations are listed in alphabetical order under the heading of the ailment. In some cases there will be more than one herbal combination listed. Under the combinations are other uses which will work as well or better as the ailment I have listed at the top. In many cases their use may be more effective than the one I have chosen.

Following Other Uses are special dietary helps that are important for the ailments listed, such as special vitamins, minerals and food that give the body extra special benefits.

The last part I have given the Orthodox Prescribed Medicine and their possible side effects.

ALLERGIES

An allergy is an overaction of the body cells to foreign materials. An allergic person may be sensitive to only one allergen, but multiple sensitivities are the rule. These could be inhalants, foods, drugs, infectious agents, contactants, physical agents or mental allergy, from which an emotional reaction may be hay fever, asthma, hives, high blood pressure, unusual fatigue and etc.

Some doctors feel that allergies are due to excessive accumulation of waste in the system due to incorrect diet, which has the effect of stirring up toxins in the body.

HERB COMBINATIONS

No. 1. _____

BLESSED THISTLE — purifies the blood, strengthens lungs
and loosens mucus and phlegm
BLACK COHOSH — relaxing to the nervous system, relieves
spasms
SCULLCAP — calming to the nerves, natural sedative, good
for headaches
PLEURISY — eliminates toxic waste through the pores,
loosens mucus in the system

No. 2 _____

GOLDEN SEAL — antibiotic for congested membranes, reduces swellings, cleans the system
CAPSICUM — stimulates the system, helps congestion, disin-
fects, increases the power of the other herbs
PARSLEY — has a tonic effect on the urinary system, increases
resistance to infection
DESERT TEA — blood purifier, decongestant, brings relief in
spasm breathing
MARSHMALLOW — helps remove mucus from lungs, heals,
soothes, and relaxes bronchial tubes.
CHAPARRAL — glandular restorer, aids lymphatic and bowels, antiseptic, tones the system
LOBELIA — stimulates, removes obstructions in the system,
acts as an expectorant, relieves spasms.
BURDOCK — blood purifier, especially lymphatic, skin and
urinary systems, removes toxic wastes through sweat
glands

OTHER USES

ASTHMA   MUCUS BUILDUP
BRONCHITIS   SINUS

COLDS   UPPER RESPIRATORY IN-
HAY FEVER   FECTIONS

SPECIAL DIETARY HELPS

A mono diet to find the allergies if its due to food. A short fast
can be useful to help clean the system and free the body of all
accumulated toxins.

VITAMIN A AND ZINC—work together to help increase
    antibodies in the system

VITAMIN B-COMPLEX — necessary for vitality, mental
    energy and nerves

VITAMINS B_{12} AND B_6 — are vital in formation of antibodies

VITAMIN C AND PANTOTHENIC ACID — are vital in the
    production of adrenal hormones which give the system an
    anti-allergic effect

VITAMIN D — helps the calcium to absorb

VITAMIN E — protects the cells against allergies

CALCIUM — works with enzymes for utilization

MINERAL — a balanced mineral tablet will help eliminate
    allergies

BEE POLLEN — Many allergies such as asthma or hay fever
    have been caused by pollen entering the respiratory sys-
    tem. Bee Pollen can build immunity by acting as a barrier
    against the inhaled pollens. Start with small amounts.

BREWER'S YEAST, GRAPE JUICE AND WHEAT GERM
    BLENDED TOGETHER — Nutrients in this blend helps
    the body strengthen its cells and walls to stop the infecting
    microbes. It's been called a natural immunity.

BROWN RICE — is called non-allergenic and its low fiber
    content is easy for the glands to absorb

FRUITS — Stone fruits (Apricots, peaches, plums, nectarines)
    will create a natural antibiotic in the blood stream to help
    build resistance and clean the system to ease sensitivity to
    allergies

GARLIC — eating fresh garlic is a natural way to help fight
    allergies such as colds and bronchial spasms

HONEY (RAW) — has been effective in the treatment of 90% of all allergies. Raw honey contains all the pollen dust and mold that causes 90% of all allergies (Carlson Wade's *Bee Pollen and Your Health*)

NUTS — high in protein, unsaturated fats, minerals and vitamins and life giving enzymes to build the blood to strengthen against allergies

AVOID — wheat products, all canned food, dairy products, citrus fruits (unless tree ripened), all sugar and salt.

ORTHODOX PRESCRIBED MEDICATION

PREDNISONE has been prescribed for hay fever. It is a cortisone-like medicine. Cortisone-type medications must be tapered off slowly to allow the body to increase its own production. Common side effects are:

Cataracts	Stomach pain
Depletion of calcium	Stomach upset
Depression	Ulcers
Indigestion	Water retention
Infections (susceptible)	

ANEMIA

Anemia is a condition in which there is a reduction in the number of circulating red blood cells. Some symptoms associated with severe anemia are weakness, vertigo, headaches, roaring in the ears, spots before the eyes, irritability, psychotic behavior, and fatigue.

Anemia often arises from recurrent infections and/or diseases involving the entire body. It could also be caused by the poor intake or absorption of nutrients or by the loss of blood during menstruation or peptic ulcers.

HERB COMBINATIONS

No. 1 _____

RED BEET — cleanses and stimulates the liver, also stimulates the spleen.

YELLOW DOCK — high in natural iron, blood purifier, and blood builder.

STRAWBERRY — high in iron, vitamin C, tones the system, helps in uric acid buildup.

LOBELIA — useful with other herbs as a powerful relaxant, removes mucus from the system.

BURDOCK — high in iron, valuable for the blood, clears the blood of harmful acids.

NETTLE — rich in iron, nourishing to the blood, tones the entire system.

MULLEIN — also very high in iron, soothing to the nerves, pain killer, and removes mucus from the system.

OTHER USES

CONVULSIONS	MULTIPLE SCLEROSIS
CRAMPS	PARKINSON'S DISEASE
ENERGY	PITUITARY GLAND
FATIGUE	SENILITY
KIDNEYS	

SPECIAL DIETARY HELPS

B-COMPLEX VITAMINS — especially B_6 and B_{12}, help to manufacture red blood cells

VITAMIN C — aids in the absorption and retention of iron

VITAMIN E — necessary for healthy red blood cells

PABA — effective in formation of blood cells, especially red blood cells

COPPER — vital to the blood along with iron

FOLIC ACID — assists in formation of blood cells, metabolism of proteins

IRON — enriches the blood, develops red blood cells

MANGANESE — works like iron in the function of red blood cells

PROTEIN — nourishes the cells and assists in metabolism

APPLES — strengthens the blood, rich in vitamins and minerals

APRICOTS — rich in iron and copper, very beneficial in anemia

BANANAS — rich in potassium

CHICKEN BREAST — complete protein

GREEN DRINK — rich in chlorophyll which is similar to human blood

DRIED BEANS AND PEAS — high in protein

EGG YOLKS — high in protein

FRUITS, FRESH, RAW

BLACKBERRIES — good blood cleanser and good for anemia

GRAINS, WHOLE — barley, millet, and buckwheat and cornmeal, natural protein and B-complex, creates bulk in the bowels, nourish the blood and cells

RAW NUTS AND SEEDS — sunflower seeds, sesame seeds, raw almonds, cashews, rich in protein, vitamins, minerals, unsaturated fats and enzymes to build the blood

VEGETABLES, DARK GREEN LEAFY — especially mustard greens, kale, swiss chard, beet greens, spinach, and collards, rich in enzymes and chlorophyll

VEGETABLES, YELLOW — rich in enzymes and works as a natural cleanser

ORTHODOX PRESCRIBED MEDICATION

A combination of IRON AND LIVER INJECTIONS are recommended for iron deficiency anemia and in certain nutritional deficiencies. Antacids given with iron compound will decrease the absorption or iron.

Possible side effects:

'Constipation   Gastrointestinal irritation
Diarrhea   Nausea

ARTHRITIS

Arthritis is defined as inflammation and soreness of the joints, usually accompanied by pain and, frequently, changes in structure. The two main types are osteoarthritis and rheumatoid arthritis. Osteoarthritis develops as a result of the constant wearing away of the cartilage in a joint. Symptoms of osteoarthritis are body stiffness and pain in the joints, during damp weather, in the morning, or after heavy exercise.

Rheumatoid arthritis affects the whole body, instead of a joint. Emotional stress usually brings on the onset of the disease. Rheumatoid arthritis destroys the cartilage and tissues in and around the joints and sometimes on the bone surface.

Symptoms include swelling and pain in the joints, fatigue, anemia, weight loss and fever.

Over 50 million Americans suffer from arthritis. It has been found that exercise is important in prevention and treatment.

HERBAL COMBINATIONS

No. 1 _____

BROMELAIN — helps in tension pain, reduces inflammation and swelling
YUCCA — cleansing agent, precursor to synthetic cortisone
COMFREY — cleans and purifies the system
ALFALFA — contains alkaloid for pain and nutrients for body strength
BLACK COHOSH — relieves pain and irritation and acid condition of blood

YARROW — acts as a blood cleanser and is soothing to the mucus, helps regulate function of the liver

CAPSICUM — stimulant, equalizes circulation, catalyst for other herbs

CHAPARRAL — dissolves uric acid accumulations and acts as an antiseptic

LOBELIA — helps remove obstructions from any part of the system, relaxant

BURDOCK — reduces swelling and deposits within joints and knuckles

CENTAURY — purifies the blood, good in muscular rheumatism

No. 2 _____

HYDRANGEA — acts like cortisone, and has the same cleaning power of chaparral

DESERT TEA — effective blood purifier, normalizes blood pressure

CHAPARRAL — contains turpentine like properties, penetrates deep into the muscles and tissue walls

YUCCA — contains saponins which break down organic wastes, like uric acid

BLACK COHOSH — natural antidote to poisons within the body

CAPSICUM — circulates through the body, increasing power of other herbs

BLACK WALNUT — contains antiseptic and healing properties, burns excess toxins

VALERIAN — counteracts poisoning, strong relaxant properties for the nerves

SARSAPARILLA — stimulating for increasing the metabolic rate, increases circulation to rheumatic joints

LOBELIA — valuable to remove obstructions from any part of the system

SCULLCAP — helps draw out uric acid, which affects the nervous system in rheumatism or neuritis

BURDOCK — blood purifier, promotes kidney function to clear the blood of harmful acids

WILD LETTUCE — has a sedative effect on the system

WORMWOOD — helps in stomach acidity, also a stomach tonic

OTHER USES

BLOOD CLEANSER	GOUT
BURSITIS	NEURITIS
CALCIFICATION	RHEUMATISM

SPECIAL DIETARY HELPS

VITAMIN A — helps to combat infection

VITAMIN B — helps in assimilating carbohydrates

VITAMIN C — (rutin and bioflavonoid) strengthens the capillary walls in the joints from breaking down and causing pain, swelling and possibly bleeding, need to take high amounts especially when taking aspirin

HISTIDINE (natural amino acid) — has anti-inflammatory properties for rheumatoid arthritis

Avoid red meat which causes uric acid build up

BRAN — two tablespoons in 8 oz. water daily helps keep colon clean

RAW FRUITS AND VEGETABLES — feed the glands and manufactures hormones

LOW SODIUM DIET — salt is toxic and causes retention of water in tissues

CALCIUM — herb combination, Comfrey, Horsetail, Oatstraw and Lobelia, is very useful

IRON, B_{12}, AND FOLIC ACID — useful in building the blood

GREEN DRINKS — contains chlorophyll which as an indirect action on bacteria, breaks down poisons

SPROUTS — contains quality protein without uric acid buildup. Full of enzymes, vitamins, minerals and energy

COD LIVER OIL — valued for vitamin D content. Lubricates
the joints and cartilage

EXERCISE — useful to help prevent and treat arthritis because
unused joints tend to stiffen

FAST FOR SEVERAL DAYS — introduce one food at a time
to determine what foods may cause the pain of arthritis.
Some doctors believe that food allergies are the cause of
most cases of arthritis. Allergies could be caused by chemicals and unnatural foods. Dr. Welsh started working with
monodiet over 57 years ago.

NATURAL FRUIT AND VEGETABLES — stay away from
acid fruits, especially lemon

ORGANIC HONEY AND BREWER'S YEAST — the 2
natural hormone foods stimulate the adrenal glands—
rejuvenating the joints, mobility of stiff fingers and limbs

PROTEIN FROM WHOLE GRAINS, NUTS AND SEEDS —
contains quality proteins, rich in vitamins, minerals and
amino acids. Nuts and seeds do not result in the formation
of excessive uric acid. Best with green vegetables—must
chew thoroughly.

TAHEEBO TEA — has helped many people eliminate arthritis.
It cleans the blood, and strengthens the body

WHEY POWDER RICH IN SODIUM — purifies the blood,
prevents calcium from depositing in the walls of the arteries

ORTHODOX PRESCRIBED MEDICATION

ASPIRIN — used in high doses (16 to 20 per day)

Common side effects:

Heartburn	Stomach pain
Nausea	Stomach ulcers
Ringing in the ears	Vomiting
Stomach bleeding	

CORTISONE — it is steroid type medicine. It is prescribed
to provide relief for inflamed areas of the body

Common side effects:

Depletion of calcium	Stomach ulcers
Depression	Susceptibility to infection
Electrolyte imbalance	Water retention
Psychosis	

BLADDER

Cystitis is an inflammation of the Urinary bladder and is common in females. It is most frequently caused by bacteria that ascend from the urinary opening or by infected urine sent from the kidneys to the bladder. Symptoms are frequent, urgent, and painful urination; pain in lower abdomen and back. Fever may occur.

HERBAL COMBINATIONS

No. 1. _____

JUNIPER BERRIES — clears mucus in bladder and kidneys, strengthens nerves, high in vitamin C
PARSLEY — high in potassium, which gives muscle tone to bladder, increases flow of urine
UVA URSI — beneficial for bladder and kidney infections, strengthens and tones urinary tract
DANDELION — very nourishing, neutralizes uric acid, opens urinary passages
CHAMOMILE — tonic, soothing to the nerves, helps elimination through the kidneys

OTHER USES

BED WETTING	URINATION PROBLEMS
DIURETIC	KIDNEY PROBLEMS
FEVERS	

SPECIAL DIETARY HELPS

VITAMIN A — fights infections
VITAMIN B-COMPLEX — helps to tone muscles of liver and
    gastro-intestinal tract
VITAMIN C — to fight infections, clears up existing infections
VITAMIN D — helps maintain stable nervous system
VITAMIN E — essential for proper liver function
PANTOTHENIC ACID — needed for healthy digestive tract
WATER, PURE — necessary to keep the cells clean
APPLE CIDER VINEGAR — cleansing and nourishing for the
    urinary tract
ASPARAGUS — contains asparagin, which acts as a stimulant
    to kidney function. It is said that the juice of asparagus
    helps break up the oxalic acid crystals in the kidneys.
BEET JUICE — cleans toxins from kidneys and restores natural
    function
CHERRY JUICE — can help stop continual urination, helps
    relieve infections
CORN SILK HERB — cleans bladder to clear infections
GARLIC — fights infection
HONEY — is hydroscopic and is able to absorb and condense
    moisture around it; will help hold the fluid in a child's
    body during sleep, may help in bed-wetting, acts as a
    sedative
JUICES, CRANBERRY AND APPLE — use cranberry,
    freshly ground with honey
LEMON JUICE — has been said to dissolve kidney stones
PARSLEY — natural diuretic, has been known to dissolve
    gravel and kidney stones
SEEDS, PUMPKIN — high in vegetable protein
SEEDS, WATERMELON — stimulates kidney action, con-
    tains cucurbocitria which is of value in dilating the large
    vessels and helps improve kidney function
TEAS, ROSE HIPS, PARSLEY, MINT, CATNIP AND
    CHAMOMILE — soothing, relaxing and healing

WATERCRESS — natural diuretic, can be used every other day altered with watermelon

ORTHODOX PRESCRIBED MEDICATION

NITROFURANTOIN is prescribed for infections of the urinary tract
Common side effects:

Chest pains	Nausea
Chills	Vomiting
Cough	Breathing problems
Diarrhea	Fever
Loss of appetite	

Less common side effects:

Dizziness	Headache
Drowsiness	Numbness

BLOOD PURIFIER

Impure blood is usually caused by poor action of the liver and bowels, faulty digestion or problems in the lymphatic glands which can be responsible for the accumulation of impurities in the blood.

The amount of toxins in the blood will vary with each person and also the degree of resistance to disease will vary with each individual. Toxemia is built up in the system to cause diseases. It is caused from eating too much of the wrong kinds of food, such as red meat, white sugar products, white flour products, coffee, cola drinks. Impurities in the air, food additives, and medicine of all kinds can also be a cause of impure blood.

HERBAL COMBINATIONS

No. 1 _____

YELLOW DOCK — nutritive tonic very high in iron, nourishes the liver and spleen

DANDELION — helps liver to detoxify poisons, blood purifier and cleanser, rich in vitamins and minerals

BURDOCK — blood purifier, promotes kidney function to clear the blood of harmful acids

LICORICE — supplies energy to the system and removes excess fluids from lungs and throat

CHAPARRAL — cleans deep into the muscles and tissue walls; cleans system of toxic wastes

RED CLOVER — eliminates toxins, tonic with valuable minerals and vitamins, with high amounts of iron and Vitamin A

BARBERRY — promotes bile in liver to clean blood, removes morbid matter from stomach and bowels

CASCARA SAGRADA — safe laxative, stimulates the secretions of the digestive system

YARROW — opens the pores freely and purifies the blood and equalizes circulation

SARSAPARILLA — contains stimulating properties, noted for increasing the metabolic rate

No. 2 _____

LICORICE — supplies energy, expectorant to expel phlegm, removes excess fluids from the lungs and throat

RED CLOVER — tonic, sedative for nervous exhaustion, antidote for cancer

SARSAPARILLA — very cleansing, glandular balance, stimulates the body's defense mechanisms

CASCARA SAGRADA — safe and effective laxative, nourishes pituitary to secrete hormones

OREGON GRAPE — purifies the blood, stimulates bile to aid digestion, tonic for all the glands

CHAPARRAL — antiseptic for deep cleansing in the tissues, potent healer, fights bacteria

BURDOCK — excellent blood purifier, removes toxic waste through the sweat glands

BUCKTHORN — stimulating effect on the liver bile, calming effect on gastrointestinal tract

PRICKLY ASH — increases the circulation, healing properties to the system

PEACH — strengthens the nervous system, stimulates urine flow, contains healing properties

STILLINGIA — removes toxic wastes from the system, stimulates the liver and glands

OTHER USES

ACNE	LYMPH GLANDS
AGE SPOTS	PANCREAS
ANEMIA	POISON IVY—OAK
ARTHRITIS	PRURITUS
BLOOD PURIFIER	PSORIASIS
BOILS	RINGWORM
CANCER	RHEUMATISM
CANKER SORES, CLEANSING	SCURVY
COLON	SKIN PROBLEMS
CONSTIPATION	SPLEEN
ECZEMA	SUGAR DIABETES
ERYSIPELAS	TETTERS
ERUPTIONS	TONSILLITIS
INFECTIONS	TUMORS
INSECT BITES	UNDULANT FEVER
JAUNDICE	URIC ACID BUILDUP
LIVER	VENEREAL DISEASE

SPECIAL DIETARY HELPS

VITAMIN A — promotes growth and repair of body tissues

VITAMIN B-COMPLEX — important in stressful situations and healthy nerves

VITAMIN C AND RUTIN — promotes healthy blood vessels

VITAMIN D — improves absorption of calcium and phosphorus in the bloodstream

VITAMIN E — dilates capillary blood vessels helping blood to flow more freely into muscle tissues

VITAMIN F — improves heart action and increases circulation

KELP — high in organic iron

LECITHIN AND NIACIN — improves appetite, digestion, assimilation, and elimination

BEET GREENS — high in iron and other minerals

CHARD — rich in iron, helps purify the blood

CHERRIES, (sour) — a natural blood cleanser

GARLIC AND CAPSICUM — cleans the blood of toxins

GREEN DRINKS — (alfalfa sprouts, spearmint, comfrey and parsley in unfiltered apple juice) cleans the blood

JUICE, CARROT AND CELERY — contains vitamins and minerals to rejuvenate the system

LEMONS AND LIMES — cleans the system of impurities, neutralizes excess acid, natural antiseptic

PARSLEY — rich in iron, cleans and builds the blood with its nutrients

SPINACH — high in iron

STRAWBERRY — helps remove metallic poisons from the blood

SPROUTS — contains live enzymes to build the blood and purify the body

WHOLE GRAINS (millet, buckwheat and barley) — contains essential protein and amino acids to withstand diseases

Avoid dead flesh in the diet for a clean blood stream

ORTHODOX PRESCRIBED MEDICATION

CYCLANDELATE called Vasodilators — increases the size of blood vessels, treats poor blood circulation

Possible side effects:

Belching	Rapid heart beat
Dizziness	Sweating
Flushing of face	Tingling sensation in face,
Headache	fingers or toes
Heartburn	Weakness
Nausea or stomach pain	

BONE KNITTER

The following herbs have been used successfully in healing bones. These herbs are combined to help nature in healing wounds and broken bones. They are also useful in healing abrasions and burns. All the herbs in this combination contain zinc. Zinc has been found essential for rapid healing.

HERB COMBINATIONS

No. 1 _____

COMFREY — heals wounds and bones, healing effect on whole system

GOLDEN SEAL — natural antibiotic with healing powers, stops infections, and contains healing vitamins and minerals

SLIPPERY ELM — strengthens the body, nutritious, draws out impurities

ALOE VERA — natural detoxicants, removes morbid matter from body, heals and protects.

OTHER USES

ABRASIONS	CUTS
BOILS	POULTICES

BROKEN BONES   WOUNDS
BURNS

SPECIAL DIETARY HELPS

VITAMIN A — helps in skin wounds along with potassium
VITAMIN B COMPLEX — provides the body with energy,
    needed daily, water-soluble and does not store in body
VITAMIN C — bioflavonoid, strengthens small blood vessels
VITAMIN D — natural blood clotting agent, strengthens
    bones, necessary for calcium assimilation
VITAMIN E — promotes and relieves healing
CALCIUM — essential in preventing breaks as well as a rapid
    healing process
DOLOMITE — bone meal, natural source of calcium, phos-
    phorus, and magnesium
ZINC — necessary for strengthening tissues, speeds healing
BROCCOLI — contains calcium, high in vitamin A
GRAINS — especially sprouted, to lessen excess mucus, and is
    rich in calcium
GREEN VEGETABLES — high content of calcium
KALE LEAVES — very high in calcium
MILK PRODUCTS — high in calcium
PARSLEY — rich in calcium and other vital minerals
PROTEIN — builds and repairs tissues
SAUERKRAUT — is rich in calcium, and is very healing and
    nourishing
SEEDS — sesame, high in iron and very high in calcium
SPROUTS — contains live enzymes quickly assimilated in the
    body
WHEY POWDER — high in sodium, dissolves any calcium
    deposits that might accumulate, the sodium in Whey Pow-
    der will help dissolve spurs on the spine

ORTHODOX PRESCRIBED MEDICATION

Drugs have a definite effect on bone fractures. Corticos-
teroid contributes to the bones being brittle. Patients who break

bones and take dolomite found that their bones healed more rapidly.

One excuse for doctors to justify prolonged use of estrogen is to prevent osteoporosis, a weakening of bones that comes with age. An intake of necessary calcium through the year would benefit.

BONES, TEETH, AND CALCIUM DEFI-CIENCY

The bones serve as a storage place for mineral salts and play an important role in the formation of blood cells. They also give shape to and support the body. Calcium deficiency can cause tooth decay, muscle cramps, nervousness, restlessness, insomnia and loss of resistance against infections, poor circulation, bronchitis and colds, among many others. High intake of meat can lead to mineral imbalance, too much phosphorus and too little calcium, which leads to calcium and magnesium deficiency and will result in loss of teeth through decay and pyorrhea. Symptoms of calcium deficiency are brittle bones, poor development of bones and teeth, dental caries, rickets, tetany, hyper-irritability, and excessive bleeding. Restlessness, insomnia, muscle cramps, back and leg pains, even asthma and hayfever are symptoms of calcium deficiency. Recently, a medical researcher says calcium deficiency is the major cause of high blood pressure.

HERBAL COMBINATIONS

No. 1 _____

COMFREY — high in calcium and phosphorus, blood cleanser, helps provide calcium and phosphorus for strong bones
HORSETAIL — rich in silica, which aids the circulation, rich in calcium, heals fractures

OAT STRAW — high in silicon, rich in calcium and phosphorus, helps prevent diseases

LOBELIA — has healing properties, removes congestion within the blood vessels

No. 2 _____

COMFREY — feeds the pituitary to help strengthen the body skeleton, high in calcium and phosphorus

ALFALFA — high in easily assimilated vitamins and minerals, alkalizer for the whole system

OAT STRAW — powerful stimulant, rich in body building materials, rich in calcium and silicon

IRISH MOSS — purifies and strengthens the cellular structure and vital fluids of the system, high in calcium

HORSETAIL — healing for fractured bones, rich in silica and selenium, strengthens the tissues

LOBELIA — strengthens the muscular action of the vessel walls to promote health

No. 3 _____

WHITE OAK — helps in reducing capillary fragility, high in B_{12}, calcium, and minerals

COMFREY — strengthens skeleton, helps in calcium and phosphorus balance

MULLEIN — nourishes and strengthens the lungs, calms the nerves, aids in keeping the glands and lymphatic system in good condition, high in iron, magnesium, potassium and sulphur

BLACK WALNUT — high in protein, contains silica, antiseptic, healing to the system

MARSHMALLOW — rich in calcium, acts as a diuretic, tonic and soothing to the nerves

QUEEN OF THE MEADOW — useful for all problems of joints, tonic, contains Vitamins A and D

WORMWOOD — helps in digestion of protein and fat, contains B complex and vitamin C

LOBELIA — healing powers with ability to remove congestion in blood vessels

SCULLCAP — strengthens the nerves, high in calcium, potassium and magnesium

OTHER USES

ACHES	HEART PALPITATIONS
ALLERGIES	HIGH BLOOD PRESSURE
ARTERIOSCLEROSIS	HORMONAL BALANCE
ARTHRITIS	HYPOGLYCEMIA
BLOOD CLOTTING	INFECTIONS
BURSITIS	INSOMNIA
CARTILAGE	JOINTS
"CHARLIE HORSES"	LACTATION
COLDS	MENSTRUAL CRAMPS
COLITIS	NERVES
CONVULSIONS	PAINS
CRAMPS	PREGNANCY
FEMALE PROBLEMS	RHEUMATISM
FLESH	TEETH
FLU	ULCERS
FRACTURES	VARICOSE VEINS
GROWING PAINS	WATER RETENTION
GOUT	WOUNDS
HEADACHES	

SPECIAL DIETARY HELPS

VITAMIN A — essential for healthy bones and teeth

VITAMIN B-COMPLEX — assists body in absorption, feeds tissues

VITAMIN B$_{12}$ — tones the muscles, acts as a nutrition stimulant

VITAMIN C — assists healing of fractures, wounds and scar tissue

VITAMIN D — essential for the absorption of calcium and phosphorus
VITAMIN E — removes scar tissue, (external and internal)
BIOFLAVONOID COMPLEX — works with vitamin C for healthy capillaries
PABA — function in metabolism of protein
CALCIUM — necessary in helping protein fibers to form a new bone
FLUORINE — preserves bones
HYDROCHLORIC ACID — helps in mineral assimilation
IODINE — necessary for development of physical growth
IRON — to build red blood cells
MAGNESIUM — increases flexibility to bones and tissues
PHOSPHORUS — assists maintenance of density in bone structure
PROTEIN — necessary in proper healing
SILICA — tones the entire system
ZINC — assists body in B-complex absorption, feeds tissues
ALMONDS — rich in calcium and protein
BEANS, PINTO — contains calcium and protein
BREWER'S YEAST — contains B vitamins, acts as a general nutrition stimulant
EXERCISE — very important
GRAINS, WHOLE — buckwheat, nourishing with proteins for building cells
GREENS, COLARD, KALE TURNIP, AND MUSTARD — high in calcium
KEFIR — helps calcium to assimilate
KELP — high in calcium
MILLET — easily digested, high in protein
SEEDS, SESAME — rich in calcium and protein
SEEDS, SUNFLOWER — moderate amounts of calcium
YOGURT — rich in calcium, easily digested
WHEY POWDER — helps in the sodium and calcium balance to prevent calcium deposits

ORTHODOX PRESCRIBED MEDICATION

MILK — is usually recommended. Chocolate interferes with calcium absorption. Chocolate milk can defeat the purpose of calcium absorption.

There has been research to show that too much meat leads to severe calcium deficiency.

Many older people lose their ability to digest milk and will develop gas, indigestion and diarrhea. (Lact-aid will help pre-digest milk sugar to eliminate this.)

CLEANSER

Herbs can be very useful in a cleansing program. Cleansing diets are very important to help rid the body of harmful accumulations of toxins. They can be caused from eating the wrong foods, air pollution, drugs, or from diseases which cause putrefaction and decay in the stomach and intestines. These germs can cause a buildup of urinary waste in the bloodstream. These excess wastes that are not eliminated can turn to solid matter or slime.

Many nutritionists recommend using herbs to empty the bowels before beginning a fast. Enemas can also be helpful. A build-up of toxic materials in the colon walls begin to decay and to form and build toxic materials which poison all areas of the body and give a general feeling of tiredness, nausea, depression, inability to do the necessary daily functions. A completely clean colon is necessary to help rid the body of diseases.

HERBAL COMBINATIONS

No. 1 _____

GENTIAN — gives strength to the system, tones the stomach, cleans blood

IRISH MOSS — high in minerals, gives strength to system, soothes tissues of lungs and kidneys

GOLDEN SEAL — cleansing action on system, kills poisons, strengthens the body

COMFREY — nourish pituitary to strengthen the body, dislodges mucus from lungs

FENUGREEK — dissolves hardened mucus, kills infections, rich in vitamins and minerals

MANDRAKE — strong glandular stimulant, supports other herbs, helps restore liver

SAFFLOWER — clears cholesterol, eliminates gastric disorders, supports adrenal glands

MYRRH — heals colon and stomach, speeds healing action, stimulates blood flow

YELLOW DOCK — purifies blood, stimulates digestion, improves liver function

ECHINACEA — slows down cleansing for safe elimination, keeps glands in working order, purifies the blood

BLACK WALNUT — balances sugar levels, burns up excess toxins in the system

BARBERRY — works on liver to help bile flow freely, removes morbid matter from stomach and bowels

DANDELION — gives nutrition to body, destroys acids in blood, eliminates toxins

ST. JOHNSWORT — tonic to system, heals obstructions of phlegm on the chest and lungs

CHICKWEED — helps curb appetite, dissolves plaque in blood vessels, strengthens stomach and bowels

CATNIP — strengthens in fatigue, sedative to nerves, rids body of bad bacteria

CYANI — stimulating tonic for the body, antiseptic to the blood

OTHER USES

ARTHRITIS   PARASITES

CANCER
COLON
CONSTIPATION
PAIN

SKIN PROBLEMS
TOXIC WASTES
TUMORS
WORMS

SPECIAL DIETARY HELPS

VITAMIN A — helps repair body tissues
VITAMIN C — detoxifies and promotes healthy blood vessels
VITAMIN D — helps maintain healthy bones and teeth
VITAMIN E — reduces uric acid, dilates capillary blood vessels helping blood flow more freely
MINERAL SUPPLEMENTS — vital to mental and physical well-being
ACIDOPHILUS — keeps intestines clean
CALCIUM — helps build blood
LECITHIN — helps maintain cell health, reduces cholesterol level in the blood
GREEN DRINKS — clean the body, contain chlorophyll
JUICES, UNFILTERED APPLE JUICE, CRANBERRY, AND GRAPE — nourishes and cleans the body
LEMON AND LIME JUICE with maple syrup, add a little garlic powder and dash of cayenne, cleans the blood
LEMON PEEL — contains rutin to strengthen the capillaries
PAPAYA — cleanse the intestines
TEAS, HERBAL — Red Raspberry, Mints, Taheebo, cleans the system
VEGETABLE BROTHS — to strengthen the body, high in potassium
WATER, PURE — cleans the system

ORTHODOX PRESCRIBED MEDICATION

MALTSUPEX — bulk forming laxatives

Common side effects:

Laxative products are overused by many people. This usually leads to dependence on laxatives. In severe cases, overuse of some laxatives has caused damage to the nerves, muscles, and tissues of the intestines and bowels. Bulk-forming laxatives often contain large amounts of sugar, carbohydrates and sodium.

COLDS

Colds are very contagious. The common cold brings about inflammation of the mucous membranes of the respiratory passages caused by viruses. It is the body's way of trying to get rid of toxins and poisons built up in the body. An acute catarrhal infection, chills, scratchy throat, sneezing, aches in the back, cough, stuffy nose, and headache.

HERBAL COMBINATIONS

No. 1. _____

ROSE HIPS — rich in vitamin C (well-known for fighting colds), helps inflamed ears, eyes, nose and throat.
CHAMOMILE — works on inflammations in ear, eyes, nose and throat and acts as a sedative
SLIPPERY ELM — removes mucus from system, soothing to lungs in colds and coughs
YARROW — purifies the blood of waste material, effective for fevers
CAPSICUM — stimulant to warm the system, helps lower fevers and increases the power of other herbs
GOLDEN SEAL — natural antibiotic, helps stop infection and heals mucous membranes
MYRRH GUM — contains antiseptic properties, used as a tonic to stimulate lungs and bronchials

PEPPERMINT — excellent for nausea, good for chills, cleans and strengthens the system

SAGE — good for excessive mucus discharge, good for fever and lungs

LEMON-GRASS — used as an anti-fever herb for flu, colds and fevers, high in Vitamin A

No. 2 _____

BAYBERRY — strong germicidal properties, stimulates mucous membranes

GINGER — induces perspiration to relieve colds, fevers; stimulates with other herbs

CLOVES — increases circulation of blood, healing properties, antiseptic

WHITE PINE — internal antiseptic, expectorant to reduce mucus secretions

CAPSICUM — helps break up congestion, increases power of other herbs, stimulant

No. 3 _____

GARLIC — antibiotic properties, acts as an expectorant, promotes sweating

ROSE HIPS — rich in vitamin C, fights colds and flu, contains vitamin P, helps infections

ROSEMARY — acts as a stimulant, helps in fatigue condition, stimulates metabolism

PARSLEY — high in vitamin A, blood builder, relaxes and nourishes run down system, contains vitamin A and C, contains calcium

WATERCRESS — high in calcium, builds immunity to infection, purifies blood, tonic

OTHER USES

BRONCHITIS   GENERAL INFECTION
CHILDHOOD DISEASES   MUCUS
EAR INFECTION   VIRAL INFECTION
FEVERS   TONSILLITIS
FLU

SPECIAL DIETARY HELPS

VITAMIN A — heals infections, high amounts for a few days
VITAMIN B6 — important in protein and carbohydrate metabolism
BIOFLAVONOIDS — necessary for healthy capillaries
VITAMIN C — to fight infection, increases resistance
VITAMIN D — improves absorption of calcium and phosphorus
VITAMIN E — reduces uric acid
CALCIUM — builds blood, sustains nerves
RUTIN — works with vitamin C for healing capillaries
FRUITS, FRESH (JUICES) — for a few days, germs are burned up and eliminated and mucus will be eliminated from the lungs
GREEN DRINKS — cleans and deodorizes the whole system
JUICE — hot lemon with honey will help open the pores and sweat
SOUP, VEGETABLE BROTH — builds the body (use every few hours)
WATER, PURE — cleans the body
WHEY DRINKS — contain lysine and quality protein, contain lactose which increases utilization of calcium magnesium, and phosphorus

ORTHODOX PRESCRIBED MEDICATION

PSEUDOEPHEDRINE — is prescribed for the relief of nasal congestion caused by colds.

High doses can cause:

Sinusitis and Hay fever   Irregular heartbeat
Hallucinations   Seizures

Common side effects:

Nervousness   Trouble in sleeping
Restlessness

Less common side effects:

Difficult or painful urination   Trembling
Dizziness or light-headedness   Troubled breathing
Headache   Weakness
Nausea or vomiting

HYDROCODONE — TUSSEND — the combination is used to relieve coughing, reduce nasal congestion, and loosen mucus and phlegm in the lungs.

Common side effects:

Dizziness   Nausea or vomiting
Drowsiness   Nervousness
Feeling faint   Restlessness
Lightheadedness   Trouble in sleeping

Less common side effects:

Constipation   Trembling
Diarrhea   Unusual increase in sweating
Difficult or painful urination Unusual weakness
Headache   Unusual fast or
Stomach pain   pounding heartbeat

When colds are suppressed with drugs, they could lead to future chronic disease. Most cold remedies have been found to be ineffective.

COLITIS

Inflammatory diseases of the colon, such as ulcerative colitis, amoebic colitis and bacillary dysentery. In the early stage there is abdominal cramps or pain, diarrhea and rectal bleeding. Instead of being absorbed by the body, water and minerals are rapidly expelled through lower digestive tract, which can cause dehydration or anemia. The cause of the disease is unknown, although there is a connection between colitis and depression or anxiety.

A healthy colon is necessary for a healthy body. When the colon is healthy, waste is removed quickly. Proper rest, exercise, emotional health, and a healthy diet is necessary for a healthy colon.

A sluggish colon could be due to improperly assimilated foods, poor eating habits, lack of exercise, lack of relaxation and emotional disturbances.

HERBAL COMBINATIONS

No. 1 _____

COMFREY — soothing to lower bowels, heals tissues, strengthens bowels

MARSHMALLOW — contains mucilage that aids the bowels, very healing

SLIPPERY ELM — soothes, draws out impurities, heals and acts as a buffer against irritations

GINGER — helps hold together all herbs, relieves gas, settles stomach

WILD YAM — relaxes the muscles of the stomach, and acts as sedative on the bowels

LOBELIA — relaxant; removes obstructions from bowels and heals

OTHER USES

INDIGESTION	INTESTINAL MUCUS
STOMACH UPSET	DIARRHEA
COLON, IRRITABLE	BOWEL PROBLEMS

SPECIAL DIETARY HELPS

VITAMINS A, E, AND B-COMPLEX — A—heals infections, B—helps restore strength to the body, C—fights infections, and E—helps eliminate poisons in the body

VITAMIN K — cold pressed oil

VITAMIN F — to restore worndown tissues

CALCIUM — dolomite, calms the nerves

IRON — to help avoid anemia

MAGNESIUM — creates a good disposition

ACIDOPHILUS — produces friendly bacteria in small intestines

BANANAS AND SWEET POTATO CASSEROLE — nourishing and soothing to the colon

BUTTERMILK — coats and soothes the stomach and colon, produces friendly bacteria in colon

COMFREY — soothing to the tissues, settles the stomach, aids absorption of iron

FASTING — can help inflammation disappear and tissues heal

FIGS — dried or tree ripened, they work upon the glands, gently prompting them by giving an emollient effect on the intestines and help bring about intestinal regularity

JUICE, FRESH ORANGE — provides vitamin C, nourishing

KEFIR — drink similar to yogurt, nourishing

KELP — helps nourish the glands

MILLET — nourishing and soothing to the digestive tract

PAPAYA — aids digestion, nourish the body

PEPSIN — soothing to the tissues, settles the stomach

RAW FOODS — should be blended until condition heals

RICE, BROWN — nourishing and easily assimilated

SPROUTS — use often when colon is healed, they act as an
   intestinal broom to keep waste matter moving along the
   intestinal tract
VEGETABLES, WHOLE — when colon is healed
WHEAT, WHOLE BREAD — helps eliminate diarrhea, provides vitamins and minerals
YOGURT — introduces friendly bacteria into the stomach,
   soothing to the colon
UNCOOKED FOODS — helps prevent accumulation of colon
   pockets, provide bulk for the diet, and prevent putrefac-
   tive fermentation.

ORTHODOX PRESCRIBED MEDICATION

   SULFASALAZINE — is a sulfa medicine. It is given to
help control inflammatory bowel disease such as colitis.

Diarrhea	Nausea
Dizziness	Sunlight sensitivity
Headache	Rash
Itching	Vomiting
Loss of appetite	

Less common side-effects:

Aching of joints and muscles
Difficulty in swallowing
Pale skin
Unexplained sore throat or fever
Unusual bleeding or bruising
Unusual tiredness or weakness
Yellowing of eyes or skin

ENERGY

   Lack of energy seems to be an epidemic in America. Poor
eating habits and lack of exercise are the chief causes. Fatigue

could be a symptom of many illnesses. One should seek for good nutrition, exercise and adequate rest. Over-eating is also a cause of lack of energy, especially white sugar products in the diet.

HERBAL COMBINATIONS

No. 1 _____

CAPSICUM — speeds up chemical reaction of herbs and equalizes blood pressure, good for circulation
SIBERIAN GINSENG — pick-up for endurance, strengthens stress defense mechanisms
GOTU KOLA — feeds brain in mental fatigue, energizing and strengthening effect to the body

OTHER USES

DRUG WITHDRAWAL   MEMORY
ENDURANCE   PICK-UP
FATIGUE   SENILITY
LONGEVITY

SPECIAL DIETARY HELPS

VITAMIN B-COMPLEX — especially B_{12} deficiency will cause abnormal fatigue, helps thinking
BIOTIN — promotes mental health
VITAMIN C — decreases the probability of blood vessel rupture and stroke, increases the aging person's ability to withstand the stress of injury and infections
VITAMIN D — necessary in tissue cell respiration and it is essential to maintain a normal basal metabolism
VITAMIN E — increases production of hormones and reduces uric acid; promotes the functions of the sexual glands
IODINE — helps thyroid to produce thyroxin, which is vital to mental energy

IRON — to enrich the blood, helps clear thinking

ALMONDS — high in protein and B-complex vitamin and calcium for energy

BEE POLLEN — contains all essential nutrients for a healthy body

BREWER'S YEAST — contains B-complex, which is the best source of enzyme-producing compunds

ENERGY DRINK — blend sunflower seeds, dates and 1 cup pure water

JUICE — tomato or vegetable with Brewer's yeast and ½ tea. kelp added as a pep-up drink

SEEDS, SUNFLOWER — protein and B-complex for energy

VEGETABLE PROTEIN — any kind will help energy

WATERCRESS — high in vitamin E and iodine, helps stimulate the brain

A daily program of food that contains a balance of vitamins, minerals, enzymes, essential fatty acids, carbohydrates and calories since the key to energy is harmony within the body

ORTHODOX PRESCRIBED MEDICATION

I have known of cases where this is prescribed by the Medical Profession.

CAFFEINE — stimulates the heart, brain and nervous system, depletes vitamins in the body, especially vitamin B, also destroys vitamin A, iron and potassium.

The caffeal content destroys the pepsin of the stomach and interferes with digestion of food and the absorption of food from the intestines.

Caffeine is an alkaloid, a vegetable poison. It is a potent central nervous system stimulant. It may lead to headache, tremors, nervousness and irritability.

Many people take coffee for energy. It is not neccesarily prescribed by doctors, but they usually don't discourage the use of it.

EYE PROBLEMS

Eye problems include cataracts, iridocyclitis, conjunctivitis, weak eyes and night blindness. Conjunctivitis is an infection of the mucous membrane that lines the eyelids. Symptoms include redness, swelling, itching and pus in the membrane. This could be caused by allergy, bacteria, virus, and air pollution.

HERB COMBINATIONS

No. 1 _____

GOLDEN SEAL — natural antibiotic for eye infections, kills poisons in the body
BAYBERRY — high in vitamin C, kills germs, stimulating to mucous membranes
EYEBRIGHT — healing, and strengthens immunity to eye complaints

No. 2 _____

GOLDEN SEAL — natural antibiotic for eye infections, kills poisons in the body
BAYBERRY — kills germs, high in vitamin C, stimulating to mucous membranes
EYEBRIGHT — heals and strengthens immunity to eye complaints
RED RASPBERRY — good for styes, astringent action helps stop discharges
CAPSICUM — stimulant, relaxant, high in vitamin A and minerals

OTHER USES

AIR POLLUTION   EYE WASH

ALLERGIES   HAY FEVER
CATARACTS   ITCHING
DIABETES   VISION (IMPROVES)
EYE INFLAMMATION

SPECIAL DIETARY HELPS

VITAMIN A — aids in vision and healthy eyes
VITAMIN B-COMPLEX — especially B6, helps prevent infection of eyes
CALCIUM — helps in preventing cataracts
VITAMIN C — detoxifying agent, heals infections
VITAMIN D — works with Vitamin A for healthy eyes
VITAMIN E — used with Vitamin A to help activate each other
CLEANSING DIET — would help improve the system and may help strengthen the eyes
JUICES, FRESH FRUIT — for severe days along with pure water to keep the bowels clear
APPLES, BLUEBERRIES, COCOANUTS — good for weak eyes
FRESH CARROT JUICE — diluted with pure water, high in vitamin A for healthy eyes
RAW POTATO JUICE — said to improve eyes
SUNFLOWER SEEDS — nourishing to the eyes, especially for weak eyes
VEGETABLES GOOD FOR WEAK EYES — beets, broccoli, cabbage, carrots, onion, turnip, collards, leaf lettuce, and watercress.

ORTHODOX PRESCRIBED MEDICATION

Antibiotics and Antivirals CHLOROPTIC, DENDRIC and HERPLEX

Possible side effects:

Stinging   Itching, redness, swelling

Blurred vision
Increased sensitivity of eyes
   to light

Pain or excess flow
   of tears

FASTING

Juice fasting helps control hunger, and helps keep blood sugar level normal while fasting. Fasting helps when we need to cleanse toxins from our body. We should eliminate mucus-forming foods from our diet. Substitute herbs instead of using prescription drugs. Fasting helps the body, physically, spiritually and mentally.

HERB COMBINATIONS

No. 1 _____

LICORICE — good for strength and quick energy, nourishes glands, inhibits growth of harmful viruses
HAWTHORNE — burns up excess fat in the body, strengthens heart, helps insomnia, calms nervous system
FENNEL — internal anesthetic, useful for gas, cramps, and mucus accumulations
BEET — stimulates and cleans the liver, nutritious, strengthens the system

OTHER USES

ADRENALS, SUPPORTS
HEART

LIVER

SPECIAL DIETARY HELPS

B-COMPLEX VITAMINS — provide the body with energy, converting carbohydrates into glucose which the body burns to produce energy
GREEN DRINKS — cleans the blood of impurities
JUICE, FRUITS — will flush impurities, contains minerals which contain alkalines to balance the acids which are in large quantity in the blood and tissues. It will cleanse the system of impurities
JUICES, VEGETABLES — a raw vegetable juice fast to cleanse out the system of toxic debris and restore the glands to health
VEGETABLE BROTH — seasoned with herbs, high in potassium which is needed for keeping the chemical balance of the fluids in the cells.

ORTHODOX PRESCRIBED MEDICATION

Sometimes water fasting is recommended. Too long a water fast can be harmful, as it removes toxic waste too fast from the system and thickens the blood to put a strain on the heart and arteries. A juice fast is much safer. It helps keep the blood stream clean, contains alkaline and helps the tissues get plenty of oxygen, keeps the bowels clean; light exercise is important.

FEMALE PROBLEMS

Recent studies have revealed that pre-menstrual tension is increased because of a lack of good nutrition and exercise. A good diet and exercise along with wise use of herbs would help alleviate the discomforts of menopause, menstrual problems, pregnancy and pre-menstrual tension.

Severe cramping during menstrual cycle could be caused by hormone imbalance. It is important to be checked by your doctor to determine any serious problems. Herbs can play an important part in female problems, whether it is cramps, menopause, pre-menstrual tension, uterine infections or pregnancy. Red Raspberry is in all the following combinations and is excellent for all female problems.

HERBAL COMBINATIONS

No. 1 _____

GOLDEN SEAL — kills infection, internal antiseptic, reduces swelling

RED RASPBERRY — high in iron, cleanses breasts for pure milk, regulates muscles in uterine contractions

BLACK COHOSH — natural estrogen, good relaxant in hysteria, neutralizes uric acid buildup

QUEEN-OF-THE-MEADOW — diuretic properties, soothes nerves helping pain in uterus

GINGER — distributes herbs to needed places, good for suppressed menstruation

MARSHMALLOW — high in calcium, healing mucous membranes, good for menstrual problems

BLESSED THISTLE — helps lactation, good for headaches, menstrual pains, stops excessive bleeding

LOBELIA — good for nerves, relaxing for painful cramps, removes obstruction

CAPSICUM — stimulates other herbs to do their job, purifies the system

No. 2 _____

RED RASPBERRY — strengthens walls of uterus, settles nausea, prevents hemorrhage

DONG QUAI — tranquilizes central nervous system, regulates menstruating, nourishes female glands

GINGER — holds herbs together, stimulating to circulation, healing properties

LICORICE — contains female estrogen, stimulates the adrenal glands, supplies energy

BLACK COHOSH — contracts the uterus, powerful sedative, tonic for nerves

QUEEN OF THE MEADOW — helps in uterine pain, diuretic, antiseptic to system

BLESSED THISTLE — internal cleanser, digestive aid, tonic to system

MARSHMALLOW — heals inflammations and prevents infections, tranquilizing system

No. 3 _____

GOLDEN SEAL — reduces swelling, kills infections, eliminates toxins

CAPSICUM — equalizes blood circulation, helps distribute herbs to where they are needed

FALSE UNICORN — useful for uterine disorders, promotes delayed menstruation, relieves depression

GINGER — binds herbs together, stimulates system, good for intestinal gas

UVA URSI — increases flow of urine, good for bladder and kidney infections

CRAMP BARK — helpful for severe menstrual or labor pains, regulates pulse, and soothing to the nerves

SQUAW VINE — antiseptic for vaginal infections, helps morning sickness, eliminates excess toxins

BLESSED THISTLE — useful for painful menstruation, helps in headaches due to female problems

RED RASPBERRY — helps reduce hot flashes, morning sickness, cramps, strengthens uterus

OTHER USES

BREAST PROBLEMS	MENSTRUAL PROBLEMS
CRAMPS	MORNING SICKNESS
HORMONE BALANCE	STERILITY

HOT FLASHES   UTERINE INFECTIONS
HYSTERECTOMY   VAGINAL PROBLEMS
MENOPAUSE

SPECIAL DIETARY HELPS

VITAMIN A — necessary in pregnancy and lactation, protects
    the body from infections and also promotes digestion
VITAMIN B-COMPLEX — especially pantothenic acid and
    PABA, help relieve nervous irritability. Brewer's Yeast
    supplements the lack of estrogen in the body due to various
    ingredients; especially needed during the middle years
    relieving the tension of all glands and nerves
VITAMIN B_1 — helps to prevent aging prematurely, protects
    the muscle of the heart; very good for improving the
    circulation
VITAMIN B_6 — decreases anxiety, heart palpitations, perspira-
    tion, and flashes and increases ability to cope with stress,
    especially in pre-menstrual tension and eases menstrual
    cramps. More energy. This vitamin stimulates the produc-
    tion of dopamine a cerebral hormone which has a calming
    effect on the nervous system. Should be taken during
    pre-menstrual week and during menstruation
VITAMIN C — helps in preventing heart attacks, assists in
    removing cholesterol from the body, blood vessels are
    strengthened, helps absorb iron, formation of red blood
    cells
VITAMIN D — great effect on the reproductive organs, impor-
    tant in preventing miscarriages and increases fertility in
    male and female
VITAMIN E — has a reducing effect on nervous sweating and
    at the same time relaxing the sympathetic nervous system
    when taken with unsaturated fatty acids (cold pressed oils)
    and with iron helps to form hemoglobin rich blood cells to
    counteract the depletion of estrogen in the body during
    menopause
DOLOMITE — Bone Meal — a great source of calcium,

phosphorus as well as other minerals, including magnesium, helps also to aid in the decreasing flow of estrogen, preventing brittle bones at the time of the "change", eases cramps also

IRON — to prevent anemia

KELP — help avoid anemia during menstrual flow. Helps the thyroid gland and helps control obesity in menopause

MANGANESE — helps in maintaining strong nerve health, helps to promote milk in pregnancy; resistance to disease, protects inside lining of the heart and blood vessels, increases activity of glandular system and assists in maintaining normal reproductive processes

ZINC — has effect on entire hormonal system, helps to absorb B complex vitamins

FRESH RAW FRUITS AND VEGETABLES — contain a quantity of hormone-like bioflavonoids which help to heal capillaries, enrich blood vessels, and help to ease leg cramps

ORTHODOX PRESCRIBED MEDICATION

ESTROGEN THERAPY

Premarin — to reduce menopause symptoms. Prolonged use can cause uterine and breast cancer and blood clots. The common side effects are:

Cramps	Mental depression
Blood pressure (increases)	Nausea
Breasts (soreness)	Skin rash
Breasts (lumps)	Swelling of ankles and feet
Eyes (yellowing)	Vaginal discharge

FITNESS

Fitness could mean the energy needed to do the necessary daily work, the ability to withstand changing eating habits, the body's stamina to avoid or overcome sickness and diseases. Exercise is very important, for it increases your capability to handle more work. It increases your heart and lung capacity and improves your mental attitude.

HERBAL COMBINATIONS

No. 1 _____

Good Athletic Formula

SIBERIAN GINSENG — stabilizes blood pressure, good for mental anxiety and nerves

HO SHOU WU — builds stamina and resistance to disease, tonic for endocrine glands

BLACK WALNUT — burns up excessive toxins and fatty material, balances sugar levels

LICORICE — stimulant for adrenal glands, supplies energy when needed, helps to maintain sugar levels

GENTIAN — high in iron, strengthens the system, stimulates the circulation, aids digestion

COMFREY — overall tonic, blood cleanser, nourishes the pituitary, high in protein

FENNEL — helps stabilize the nervous system and acts as an internal anesthetic

BEE POLLEN — strengthens and builds the system, increases work capacity, an energizing food, helps build resistance to stress and colds, influences the adrenal hormones, athletes claim championship performances

BAYBERRY — rejuvenates the adrenal glands, cleans the blood stream, removes waste

MYRRH — gives vitality and strength to the digestive system, a cleansing and healing herb

PEPPERMINT — sedative to the stomach, strengthens the
    bowels, aids digestion
SAFFLOWER — removes hard phlegm from the system, good
    for the liver and gall bladder
EUCALYPTUS — antiseptic properties, potent but safe,
    purifies
LEMONGRASS — stimulates heart, calms nerves, tightening
    action on tissues
CAPSICUM — stimulates the system, disinfectant to body,
    equalizes blood circulation

OTHER USES

DIETS   FASTING
ENDURANCE   GLANDS
ENERGY   STRENGTH

SPECIAL DIETARY HELPS

VITAMIN B-COMPLEX — especially B_1, B_3, B_{12} and B_{15}.
    Thiamine depletion is caused by excessive amounts of
    sugar, smoking and alcohol, B_3 works in the enzymatic
    breakdown of sugar in the body's energy cycle
VITAMIN C — for stress and alertness, helps in fatigue
VITAMIN E — improves stamina and lung control of oxygen
AMINO ACIDS, ESSENTIAL — necessary to healthy cells in
    the body
MAGNESIUM — essential for effective nerve and muscle
    function
BEE POLLEN — increases endurance
BREWER'S YEAST — concentrated live food with B vitamins
    and protein, increases the action of vitamin E
FRUITS — increases energy, apricots, cantaloupe, guava,
    papayas, peaches

ORTHODOX PRESCRIBED MEDICATION

AMPHETAMINES — BENZEDRINE and METHAD-

RINE often called "uppers" and "pep pills", have been used by athletes and diet conscious persons. It increases heart rate, blood sugar, muscle tension, and gives a sense of well-being. The extra energy is borrowed from the body's reserves. When the drug's action has worn off, the body pays for it in fatigue and depression. This creates the desire for more of the drug.
Possible side effects:

Psychic dependence
Physical deterioration due to hyperactivity and lack of appetite
Prolonged dosage can create induced psychotic condition of paranoia
and schizophrenia

FLU

The flu is a highly contagious disease caused by a virus, usually accompanied by fever, aches, pains, inflammation of respiratory mucous membranes, easily spread by sneezing and coughing. It is also accompanied by chills, sore throat, headache, and swollen lymph nodes. The complications are pneumonia, sinus infection, and ear infection.

HERBAL COMBINATIONS

No. 1 _____

GINGER — removes congestion, relieves headaches, soothes
    sore throat, binds herbs together
CAPSICUM — stimulating to warm the system, helps reduce
    fever
GOLDEN SEAL — destroys germs, strong antibiotic
LICORICE — removes excess fluid from lungs, relieves cough-
    ing, sore throat, helps supply energy

OTHER USES

NAUSEA   MOTION SICKNESS
VOMITING   MORNING SICKNESS

SPECIAL DIETARY HELPS

VITAMIN A — is important for health of the lining of the throat
    and nose, when flu hits take 25,000 units
VITAMIN B-COMPLEX — good for stress
VITAMIN C — healing and fighting infections
PANTOTHENIC ACID — necessary for proper digestion
PROTEIN — needed for repair of tissue destroyed by fever
FLUIDS AND JUICES — cleans body of toxins, provides
    strength
GRAPEFRUIT — equal part pure water and grapefruit juice
    will ease the flu
WATER — drink lots of pure water
ENCOURAGE PERSPIRATION — helps eliminate virus and
    congestion, hot lemon and honey will produce perspira-
    tion
LETTUCE, GREEN, LEAFY AND FRESH — boil in lots of
    pure water, drink six ounces each day
FASTING — helps in flu, quickest way to cleanse the body of
    impurities

ORTHODOX PRESCRIBED MEDICATION

INFLUENZA VIRUS VACCINE — TRIVALENT
Possible side effects:

Fever, malaise   Deaths occur primarily among
Myalgia within 6-12 hours   chronically ill or those
Possible paralysis   over 65 years of age

GLANDS

All glands are vital to a healthy system. They need to be nourished especially with minerals. Vitamins and minerals play an important part in supplying the body with the raw material to manufacture its own hormones which are the secretions of the glands.

These hormones are essential secretions affecting the whole system, and are connected with growth and health. The glands depend on the necessary intake of the vital vitamins and minerals for their efficient functioning. The thyroid gland stimulates all of the cells of the body. The hormones from the thyroid are powerful and need to be kept under exact control.

Lack of iodine is a common cause of trouble. Diseases or drugs can effect the thyroid, also stress or hereditary defect.

HERBAL COMBINATIONS

No. 1

KELP — contains iodine which strengthens and reactivates the glands, strengthens blood and central nervous system
DANDELION — stimulates glands, increases activity of liver, tonic, nutritious
ALFALFA — increases glandular secretions, nourishes glands

No. 2

LOBELIA — removes obstruction in system, healing, relaxes nerves
MULLEIN — contains harmless narcotic properties, calming to the nerves

OTHER USES

ASTHMA   PETS (VITAMINS AND MINERALS)

BREASTS   PITUITARY
BRONCHITIS   PLEURISY
CROUP   PNEUMONIA
LIVER   RHEUMATISM
LYMPH CONGESTION   THYROID
MUCUS   TONSILLITIS
NERVES   TUBERCULOSIS
PAIN

SPECIAL DIETARY HELPS

VITAMIN A — healing vitamin, rejuvenates the glands, repairs damaged tissues

VITAMIN B-COMPLEX — necessary for metabolism of the extra carbohydrates and protein, helps replenish nutrition to glands

VITAMIN C — healing vitamin, protects the glands, helps glands to become nutritionally replenished

VITAMIN E — increases production of hormones

CALCIUM — assists all metabolic functions to perform efficiently

CHLORINE — acts in formation of glandular hormones, helps in metabolism

IODINE — aids thyroid gland, promotes metabolism, prevents goitre

IRON — nourishes the glands

MAGNESIUM — stimulates the glands

MANGANESE — increases gland secretion

PHOSPHORUS — promotes secretion of hormones

POTASSIUM — increases glandular secretions

SILICON — stimulates and feeds the glands

ZINC — necessary for synthesis of new body protein

ALFALFA SPROUTS — full of enzymes, nourishing to the glands

AVOCADO — gland food, use with olive oil

BROCCOLI — feeds weak glands involved in digestion of food

DATES — nourishing food for glands

FIGS (TREE-RIPENED) — medicine for the glands, supplies nutrients

FLUIDS — fresh pure water, fresh fruit and vegetable juices

NUTS, RAW ALMOND AND CASHEW — supplies protein, needed daily for the cells

OLIVE OIL — lubricates the system, supplies vitamins

PARSLEY — cleans the glands, nourishes

PROTEIN (NOT RED MEAT) — to replace muscle tissue and build cells

RAISINS — nourishes the glands

RICE AND BRAN — feeds the glands and cells

RYE — good for the glands, high in protein

SEEDS — pumpkin, squash, sunflower, and sesame, seeds are gland foods

VEGETABLES — green, dark, leafy

YAMS — gland food

ORTHODOX PRESCRIBED MEDICATION

LIOTRIX or THYROGLOBULIN — thyroid hormone

Possible side effects:

Constipation	Rapid pulse
Chest pain	Shortness of breath
Hives	Tiredness
Listlessness	Unusual weight gain
Muscle aches	

HEART

Heart attacks are the leading cause of death in the U.S. Many Americans have coronary artery disease, which is characterized by a narrowing of the blood vessels that nourish the heart muscle. The narrowing of the vital coronary vessels may progress for many years before any adverse effects are evident. In many instances a heart attack is the first overt sign of the disease.

HERBAL COMBINATIONS

No. 1 _____

HAWTHORNE — strengthens the heart, helps prevent blood
    clot near heart, high in minerals
CAPSICUM — takes other herbs to the heart, circulation
GARLIC — kills infection, heart palpitation, lowers blood
    pressure, beneficial to blood vessels

OTHER USES

ADRENAL	HARDENING OF ARTERIES
ARTERIOSCLEROSIS	IRREGULAR HEART BEAT
ANXIETY	LIVER
CIRCULATION	PAIN
CHOLESTEROL	SHOCK
FATIGUE	VARICOSE VEINS

SPECIAL DIETARY HELPS

VITAMIN B-COMPLEX — especially B_1, B_{15}, necessary to
    maintain the health of the arteries
VITAMIN C — nourishes the capillaries
VITAMIN D — relaxes nerves, helps calcium absorb
VITAMIN E — needed as an anti-coagulant to reduce arterial
    clots and to get oxygen to the blood
VITAMIN F — increases circulation
VITAMIN K — aids blood coagulation and controls consis-
    tency of blood
CALCIUM — calms nerves, strenthens heart muscles
LECITHIN — helps eliminate cholesterol
MAGNESIUM — alkalizes the system, aids blood circulation

PHOSPHORUS — helps in acid, alkaline balance
POTASSIUM — vital in preventing heart attacks (combined
    with magnesium)
DIET, CLEANSING — to clean out the arteries
FRUITS, FRESH — live enzymes, vitamins and minerals to
    nourish the heart
GRAINS, WHOLE — contains B-complex vitamin, minerals,
    enzymes and amino acids to the gland which helps to
    maintain a healthful blood cholesterol level. The hor-
    mones feed the heart muscles to send oxygen to the cir-
    culatory system
OILS, COLD PRESSED — it sends a natural anti-oxidant
    hormone to the heart and boosts the heart-blood circula-
    tion
PROTEIN — vegetable is better quality, does not leave uric
    acid build-up
Use honey, pure maple syrup, malt sugar, date sugar instead of
    white sugar
OLIVES — rich in potassium
POTASSIUM SOUP — potato peelings, celery, onions, car-
    rots, parsley. Cook and strain

ORTHODOX PRESCRIBED MEDICATION

NITROGLYCERIN — it is prescribed to improve the
supply of blood and oxygen to the heart. Also to relieve pain
and/or prevent heart attacks.

Possible side effects:

Headache   Vomiting
Dizziness   Skin rash
Weakness   Flushing
Nausea

PROCAINAMIDE — prescribed to restore irregular
heartbeats to a normal rhythm and to slow an overactive heart.

Common side effects:

Diarrhea	Nausea
Loss of appetite	Vomiting

Less common, but possible side effects:

Fever	Pains with breathing
Itching	Skin rash
Joint pain or swelling	

Rare but possible side effects:

Mental confusion	Unexplained fever and
Mental depression	sore throat
Hallucinations	Unusual bleeding or bruising

HIGH BLOOD PRESSURE

Hypertension is a condition in which the person has a higher blood pressure than is judged to be normal. High blood pressure is the body's extensive measure to cope with functions of the body, such as toxemia, kidney problems, glandular disturbances, degenerative changes in arteries, overweight or emotional problems.

With high blood pressure, there is a thickening of the blood from catarrhal and excess matter loading the circulatory system.

High blood pressure is usually characterized by flushed complexion, over-weight, and discomfort. Some doctors feel it is a result of improper living habits which cause a run-down condition of the body.

High and low blood pressure are both due to malfunction of the circulatory system.

Cholesterol must be eliminated from the system to help the blood to flow more easily.

Stress is a factor in causing high blood pressure and should be controlled.

HERBAL COMBINATIONS

No. 1 _____

CAPSICUM — stimulates the system and the ingredient of garlic reduces the dialated blood vessels

GARLIC — antibiotic, opens up the blood vessels and reduces blood pressure in hypertension

No. 2 _____

GARLIC — helps stabilize blood pressure, purifies the system

CAPSICUM — carries the herbs where needed, natural stimulant

PARSLEY — high in iron, natural diuretic, helps resist infection

GINGER — helps bind the herbs together, removes excess waste from the body

SIBERIAN GINSENG — stabilizes blood pressure, hormone regulator

GOLDEN SEAL — antiseptic, cleans any infection, controls secretions

OTHER USES

CIRCULATION	INFECTIONS
COLDS	LOW BLOOD PRESSURE
FLU	NERVES
HIGH BLOOD PRESSURE	STRESS
HYPERTENSION	TENSION

SPECIAL DIETARY HELPS

VITAMIN A — builds the immune system

VITAMIN B-COMPLEX — high potency, calms the nerves and helps build the blood

VITAMIN C — strengthens the blood vessels

VITAMIN E — dialates the blood vessels, could temporarily elevate blood pressure, small amount to start

BIOFLAVONOIDS — helps maintain the health of the blood vessels, and capillaries

CALCIUM — a deficiency has been found to be a major cause of high blood pressure

CHOLINE — (found in lecithin) — prevents fats from accumulating in the liver and assists the movement of fats into the cells

MAGNESIUM — helps the nervous system and promotes sleep

LECITHIN — breaks up cholesterol and allows it to pass through the arterial wall, helping to prevent artherosclerosis

MANGANESE — necessary for proper nutrition, activates other minerals

POTASₒIUM — will cause the body to excrete more sodium

RUTIN — to strengthen capillaries

SULPHUR — promotes bile secretions, purifies the system

TYROSINE (NATURAL AMINO ACID) — experiments in Israel have shown to help reverse high blood pressure

ZINC — influences acid-alkaline balance in body

BROCCOLI — good for high blood pressure

BUCKWHEAT — complete protein equal to animal protein

CANTALOUPE — full of vitamins and minerals, has been recommended for high blood pressure

DIET, LOW SALT

DIET, RICE AND FRUIT — recommended to help clear out the system

EXERCISE — is important to keep the circulation system healthy

GARLIC — contains sulphur and manganese, helps cholesterol and cleans the blood vessels

PARSLEY — natural diuretic, full of vitamins and minerals

PINEAPPLE — regulation of the glands and is valuable for high blood pressure

RICE, WILD — high in vitamins and minerals and low in fat

STRAWBERRIES — cleans the blood of harmful toxins

TEA, TAHEEBO — cleans the blood, strengthens the body

TOMATOES — natural antiseptic and protects against infection, helps in high blood pressure

WATERMELON — cleans out the system. The seeds contain cucurbocitrin, which dilates the capillaries, the tiny blood vessels. This relieves pressure on the large blood vessels.

ORTHODOX PRESCRIBED MEDICATION

RESERPINE AND HYDRALAZINE

Medicines called Antihypertensives — they are prescribed to treat high blood pressure. They are also sometimes used to treat certain mental and emotinal conditions.

Common side effects:

Drowsiness or fainting	Mental depression
General feeling of body discomfort or weakness	Nervousness
Headache	Vivid dreams or nightmares
Impotence or decreased sexual interest	

Less common side effects:

Black, tarry stools	Skin rash
Chest pain	Stiffness
Bloody vomit	Swelling of feet or lower legs
Numbness	Swelling of lymph glands
Shortness of breath	

HYPOGLYCEMIA

Hypoglycemia is a condition where there is a deficiency of sugar in the blood or low-blood sugar, in other, words a condition in which the glucose in the blood is abnormally low. The symptoms are: fatigue, restlessness, malaise, marked irritability and weakness. In severe cases, mental disturbances, delirium, coma and possibly death can occur.

HERBAL COMBINATIONS

No. 1 _____

LICORICE — supplies quick energy to weakened systems
SAFFLOWER — helps the adrenal glands to produce more ad   alin and encourages the pancreas to manufacture natural insulin
DANDELION — destroys acids in the blood, helps in anemia, balances blood in all nutritive salts
HOR° ERADISH — contains antibiotic action, stimulates and cleans the system

No. 2 _____

SOY PROTEIN — high in protein, gives strength to the system, high in lecithin
CAPSICUM — stimulating to system, cleans body, high in nutritious vitamins and minerals
RED CLOVER — clears mucus, cleans system of impurities, fights infection

OTHER USES

ADRENAL GLANDS   LIVER
ANEMIA   PANCREAS
ENERGY   WEAKENED SYSTEM

SPECIAL DIETARY HELPS

VITAMIN A — gives strength and vitality, promotes healthy feeling

VITAMIN B-COMPLEX — helps in nervous exhaustion, anti-stress vitamin helps normalize sugar level

VITAMIN B_6 — helps build adrenal glands

VITAMIN B_{12} — helps restore liver function

VITAMIN C — has been said to prevent low blood sugar attacks if taken daily

VITAMIN E — helps in the oxygenation of cells, necessary when sugar levels are low

PANTOTHENIC ACID — stimulates adrenal gland

MAGNESIUM — diabetics require more than the normal dose, necessary for the nerves

CHROMIUM — is essential to the utilization of glucose

BREWER'S YEAST — B compelx to feed the cells and nerves

FREQUENT SMALL MEALS — Provides quick energy

NUTS — good source of protein and unsaturated fats as well as vitamins and minerals

SEEDS — high in protein, high in calcium and very nutritious, high in amino acid balance that enhances utilization

NATURAL CARBOHYDRATES — needed in small quantities to provide energy, excess stores in the body as fat

WHOLE GRAINS, NUTS, SEEDS — high quality protein

VEGETABLES — fresh for enzymes, vitamins and minerals

ORTHODOX PRESCRIBED MEDICATION

There is no known prescribed medication for hypoglycemia. There are no known drugs to specifically elevate the blood sugar level.

GLUCAGON — belongs to the medicines called hormones. This is an emergency medicine to treat severe hypoglycemia. It is used by injection if the patient becomes unconscious as a result of hypoglycemia.

In many cases high animal protein is recommended. This could lead to uric acid build up in the system.

Side effects could cause vomiting.

Glucagon is not effective for much longer than 1½ hours and is only used until the patient is able to swallow liquids.

INFECTIONS

The condition in which the body or part of it is invaded by microorganisms or virus. The symptoms of infection are those of inflammation, swelling, and soreness. To keep infections from remaining in the system, some doctors suggest encouraging perspiration, activating the kidneys, and opening the bowels, because fevers tend to dry up the bowels. Take natural laxative and protein foods, for protein of animal origin are contra-indicated in infectious disease. Also give raw fruits and vegetable juices while fever lasts.

HERBAL COMBINATIONS

No. 1 _____

(especially for hypoglycemia)
ECHINACEA — purifies blood, detoxifies, increases resistance to infections
YARROW — blood cleanser, eliminates waste, equalizes circulation, strengthens system
MYRRH — antiseptic properties, vitality and strengthens the system
CAPSICUM — stimulant to the system, helps circulation, cleanses the system

No. 2

ECHINACEA — blood purifier, natural antibiotic, gland cleanser, builds immunity to infection

GOLDEN SEAL — antibiotic, kills poisons in system, reduces swellings, valuable for all catarrhal conditions

YARROW — blood cleanser, opens pores to permit perspiration, eliminates impurities and reduces fevers

CAPSICUM — reduces dialated blood vessels in chronic congestion, stimulant, disinfectant

No. 3

GOLDEN SEAL — acts as a natural antibiotic, reduces swelling, heals mucous membranes

BLACK WALNUT — burns up excess toxins, kills infections, tones up the system

MARSHMALLOW — removes difficult phlegm from system; heals, soothes and neutralizes

LOBELIA — relaxing to the system, removes obstruction from system, neutralizes infections

PLANTAIN — neutralizes poisons, acts as a laxative, soothing to whole system

BUGLEWEED — helps reduce fluid discharges, relieves pain, relaxes the body

OTHER USES

BREASTS, INFECTION	LUNGS
COLDS	MEASLES
CONTAGIOUS DISEASES	MUMPS
EARACHE	RHEUMATISM
FEVERS	SCARLET FEVER
FLU	SINUS INFECTION
GANGRENE	THROAT, SORE
GLANDS, INFECTED, SWOLLEN	TONSILLITIS
INFECTIONS	TYPHOID FEVER

SPECIAL DIETARY HELPS

VITAMIN A — large doses for a short period, promotes healing, fights infections

VITAMIN B-COMPLEX — infections can cause depletion of B-complex, necessary to help maintain energy

VITAMIN B6 — acts as a natural antihistamine, defends body against infections

VITAMIN C — massive dose helps fight early infection, helps in allergy related infections

VITAMIN E — works with vitamin A to promote healing, heals infections, removes scar tissue

BIOFLAVONOIDS — strengthens capillaries, helps heal infections

ZINC — speeds up the healing of external and internal wounds

BROTH, VEGETABLE — high in potassium, builds health

FRUITS, FRESH — helps remove impurities from the blood

FRUITS, FRESH JUICES — purifies the system, builds the body

WATER, PURE — cleans the system of poisons

WATERCRESS, WILD — eaten regularly will help build immunity to colds, catarrhs, and infectious diseases

ORTHODOX PRESCRIBED MEDICATION

ANTIBIOTICS — Penicillin, Tetracycline or Erythromycin

Common side effects:

Cramps or burning of stomach	Nausea
	Sore mouth or tongue
Diarrhea	Vomiting
Increased sensitivity to sunlight	Hives
	Itching
Itching of the rectal or genital area	Swelling of face and ankles
	Blood in the urine

INSOMNIA

Insomnia is the inability to sleep, because it is prematurely ended or interrupted by periods of wakefulness. It could be a symptom of a disease, but it is not a disease in itself. Anxiety and pain are the most frequent causes of insomnia. Some people with ailments such as asthma or heart disease may be unable to sleep for fear of suffocation. Avoid caffeine drinks.

HERBAL COMBINATIONS

No. 1 _____

VALERIAN — relaxant, sedative, tonic, tranquilizer with refreshed feeling
SCULLCAP — feeds the nerves, controls nervous disorders, relaxes the mind
HOPS — produces sleep, helps restlessness, acts as a nervine for insomnia

OTHER USES

CONVULSIONS   PALSY
HEADACHES   RELAXANT
HYPERACTIVITY   STRESS
NERVES

SPECIAL DIETARY HELPS

VITAMIN B-COMPLEX — relaxing to the nerves
VITAMIN B$_6$ — essential to break tryptophan down into niacin
VITAMIN B$_{15}$ — improves the body's ability to withstand stressful conditions
TRYPTOPHAN (ESSENTIAL AMINO ACID) — it has been used for psychiatric problems, to induce sleep and to quiet the nervous system

CALCIUM — calms the nerves, gives strength
CHOLINE — assists in transmission of nerve impulses
FOLIC ACID — metabolism of proteins
BATHS, WATER — help relax
EXERCISE — vigorous morning exercise causes the release of
    a hormone called prostaglandin which promotes sleep 12
    hours later
JUICE, CELERY — promotes sleep
TEA, CHAMOMILE — produces restful sleep, but avoid a
    heavy meal in the evening

ORTHODOX PRESCRIBED MEDICATION

PHENOBARBITOL or CARBROMAL — medicines called central nervous system depressants. They are given to treat insomnia or sleeplessness.

Possible side effects:

Dizziness — caused by low calcium levels	Unusual sore throat and fever
Light headedness	Unusual bleeding or bruising
Drowsiness	Unusual excitement
"Hangover" effect	Tiredness
Swelling of eyelids, face or lips	Weakness
	Slow heart beat

KIDNEYS

The function of the kidneys is to excrete urine which contains the end products of metabolism, and to help regulate the wastes, electrolyte and acid base content of the blood. Nephritis is an inflammation of the kidneys. Avoid foods that contain oxalic acid, caffeine, theobromine, and caffeal (more concentrated in decaffeinated coffee). They are irritating to the kidneys. Coffee, chocolate and excessive meat should be avoided.

HERBAL COMBINATIONS

No. 1 ————————————————————————

GOLDEN SEAL — antiseptic for kidneys, helps kidneys eliminate toxins, healing

JUNIPER — antiseptic to kidneys. Eliminates mucus from the kidneys, high in Vitmain C

UVA URSI — acts as solvent to urinic calculii deposits, strengthens urinary tract

PARSLEY — nutritional to the kidneys, tones up the urinary system, builds resistance

GINGER — enhances effectiveness of other herbs, cleans the kidneys

MARSHMALLOW — helps remove phlegm from kidneys, soothing to urinary tract, nutrition

LOBELIA — helps clear obstructions from the system, relaxing, healing

OTHER USES

BED WETTING   DIURETIC
BLADDER   URINARY PROBLEMS

SPECIAL DIETARY HELPS

VITAMIN A — necessary to keep the kidneys healthy

VITAMIN B6 — important for proper functioning of the pancreas

VITAMIN C — helps keep the kidneys healthy and in good repair

VITAMIN E — helps clear up kidney problems

LECITHIN — helps purify the kidneys

MANGANESE — essential for proper nutrition, activates other minerals

MAGNESIUM — valuable to the nervous system

POTASSIUM — stimulates the liver, converts sugar into energy

ZINC — has an effect on acid-alkaline balance of the system. Necessary to keep the kidneys healthy

APPLES — contain malic and tartaric acids, which helps keep digestion and the liver healthy

GRAPES — the alkaline in grapes helps to decrease the acidity of the uric acid and to eliminate it from the system, thus helping the kidneys

JUICES — cherry and apple and cranberry

LEMON JUICE — in pure water, ½ lemon at a time, a natural antiseptic, destroys bacteria

LIQUIDS — avoid sweet drinks like soda pop, coffee, tea, chocolate and white sugar products and starches. These could cause inflammation of the lining membranes of the kidneys.

PARSLEY — natural diuretic, rich in minerals and vitamins and is valuable for nephritis

PEARS — helps in inflammation of the kidneys such as nephritis

SOUP — using asparagus, celery, spinach and parsley, use an herb seasoning

WATERCRESS — very high in Vitamin C, has been recommended for kidney disorders

WATERMELON — well known for correcting kidney problems, the seeds contai· cucurbocitrin which has the effect of dialating the capillaries, relieving pressure on the large blood vessels

ORTHODOX PRESCRIBED MEDICATION

PENICILLINS for Nephritis (Kidney infections)

Possible side effects are:

Hives

Itching

Rash

Wheezing

Diarrhea

Nausea

Vomiting

Blood in urine

Passage of large amounts of
    light colored urine

Swelling of face and ankles

Troubled breathing

Unusual tiredness or
    weakness

LIVER

The liver manufactures digestive enzymes and acts as a filter between the intestines and the heart. It helps detoxify the poisons which are taken into the system. The liver controls and regulates the quantity, the quality and the use of the foods we eat. It regulates the appetite, for in the case of hepatitis, one of the first signs is loss of appetite.

The liver has a vital influence on the emotions of the body. A healthy liver will help in endurance, patience, and perseverance. A sluggish liver, with accumulated toxins can cause nausea, headaches, indigestion, loss of appetite, constipation, pain on the right side, cold sweats, and jaundice.

Liver problems usually involve congestion, hepatitis, and sluggishness. The liver is a powerful detoxifying organ, breaking down toxic materials, and producing bile. The three most common liver diseases are: liver cancer, cirrhosis, and hepatitis.

HERBAL COMBINATIONS

No. 1 _____

RED BEET — nutritious for liver function, helps correct liver
    disease

DANDELION — stimulates the liver, detoxifies poisons, clears liver obstructions

PARSLEY — cleans liver of toxic wastes, tones the body, nutritious to build system

HORSETAIL — rich in vitamins and minerals, aids in circulation, builds and tones the body, diuretic

LIVERWORT — vitamin K and other nutrients important to strengthen the liver, heals damaged liver

BIRCH — natural properties for cleansing the blood, high content of vitamins and minerals

LOBELIA — used as an antidote, removes obstructions from the body, sedative

BLESSED THISTLE — general tonic to system, stimulates liver bile, purifies blood

ANGELICA — helps eliminate toxins in liver and spleen, tonic for mental and physical harmony

CHAMOMILE — destroys toxins in liver, healing properties, aid for insomnia

GENTIAN — stimulates liver, high in iron, strengthens the system, aids digestion

GOLDEN ROD — stimulates circulation, kidney function, strengthens system

No. 2

BARBERRY — corrects liver secretions (causes the bile to flow more freely)

GINGER — works as a diffusive stimulant

CRAMP BARK — good for congestion and hardening of the liver

FENNEL — helps move waste material out of the body

PEPPERMINT — cleans and strengthens the entire body

WILD YAM — good for hardening and blocking of the liver

CATNIP — used as a tonic to strengthen the liver and gall bladder

OTHER USES

AGE SPOTS   KIDNEYS
CLEANSING   PANCREAS
GALL BLADDER   SPLEEN

SPECIAL DIETARY HELPS

VITAMIN A — promotes digestion and food assimilation
VITAMIN B-COMPLEX — Provides amino acids, strengthens
    system
VITAMIN B$_6$ — promotes digestion and elimination
VITAMIN B$_{12}$ — helps in digestion, assimilation and elimina-
    tion
VITAMIN C — detoxifying properties, heals infections
VITAMIN D — stored in the liver for all over healthy feeling
VITAMIN E — helps reduce uric acid
VITAMIN K — helps liver function to properly absorb food
MAGNESIUM — stimulates the liver
ZINC — aids digestion, helps the acid, alkaline balance
SULPHUR — aids the liver in bile secretion
CHOLINE — helps detoxify fatty and congested liver and
    assists liver function
INOSITOL — helps prevent gall bladder problems, helps pre-
    vent fatty liver
METHIONIME — (amino acid) necessary for liver regenera-
    tion, removes poisonous wastes from the liver and protects
    the liver
VEGETABLES — artichokes, cauliflower, collards, endives,
    green peppers, pomegranate, quince, raspberries, straw-
    berries, and tangerines
FRUIT JUICES, FRESH — cleans the liver, strengthens the
    system
FRUITS — apples, cherries, cranberries, gooseberries, plums,
    pomegranate, quince, raspberries, strawberries and
    tangerines
LIVER-PANCREAS STIMULANT — nutmeg - ½ teaspoon,

cardamon - pinch, pure water - 1 cup hot — this helps the
pancreas to release juices and will rebuild the liver
CARROT JUICE — cleans and nourishes the liver
DANDELION TEA — cleansing for the liver
GARLIC — helps detoxify bacteria in the intestines
GRAINS, BEANS — protein, helps in the formation of impor-
tant enzymes, hormones and disease, fighting antibodies
GRAPES — helps liver disorders, jaundice and stimulates bile
flow
WATERCRESS AND PARSLEY — relieves liver inflamma-
tion
OLIVE OIL IN ORANGE OR LEMON JUICE — helps dis-
solve hard bile
Avoid sugar, starches, fats, eggs, cream, spices, alcohol,
chocolate and caffeine drinks to bring quicker results

ORTHODOX PRESCRIBED MEDICATION

CHOLESTYRAMINE — removes bile acids from the
body with liver problems, where there is too much bile acid in
the body.
Common side effect:

Constipation

Less common:

Severe stomach pain   Unusual loss of weight
Nausea and vomiting

KANAMYCIN — antibiotics used to help lessen the
symptoms of hepatic coma, a complication of liver disease.
Possible side effects:

Irritation or soreness of the   Some loss of hearing
mouth or rectal area   Clumsiness
Nausea   Dizziness
Vomiting   Excessive thirst

LOWER BOWELS

An underactive bowel can cause toxic wastes to be absorbed through the bowel wall and into the bloodstream—which can cause them to deposit in the tissues. As toxins accumulate in the tissues, they can cause cell destruction. Other problems can arise, such as poor digestion, fatigue, poor circulation and many other ailments because of improper diet and impacted bowels.

HERBAL COMBINATIONS

No. 1 _____

CASCARA SAGRADA — restores tone to relaxed bowel, cleans and nourish system

BUCKTHORN — stimulates the bile, good for constipation, calming on gastrointestinal tract

LICORICE — mild laxative, supplies energy, beneficial to the liver

CAPSICUM — stimulates the bowels, internal cleanser, increases the power of all the other herbs

GINGER — internal stimulant, holds herbs together, settles the stomach.

BARBERRY — promotes bile in liver, calming for the nerves, cleansing for the system

COUCH GRASS — antibiotic, tonic, cleans the urinary tract, diuretic

RED CLOVER — cleans mucus from the system, fights infection, high in iron and minerals

LOBELIA — removes obstructions from all parts of body, relaxant, healing to bowels

No. 2 _____

CASCARA SAGRADA — stimulates the gall bladder, helps liver problems, stimulates adrenal glands

RHUBARB — reduces blood pressure, good for chronic diarrhea, reduces inflammations

GOLDEN SEAL — strong antibiotic, relieves inflammations, strengthens liver, healing

CAPSICUM — increases blood circulation, distributes herbs throughout the system

GINGER — binds other herbs together, soothing to nervous system, helps intestinal gas

BARBERRY — strong antiseptic properties, blood cleanser, removes morbid matter from stomach and bowels

LOBELIA — draws mucus congestion from the system, relaxant

FENNEL — relieves gas, colic and cramps, nourishes the system

RED RASPBERRY — good for stomach problems, strengthens the system, supplies nutrients

OTHER USES

BAD BREATH	CONSTIPATION
BOWEL DISCOMFORTS	CROUP
CLEANSING	DIARRHEA
COLITIS	INTESTINAL MUCUS
COLON	PARASITES

SPECIAL DIETARY HELPS

VITAMIN A — promotes digestion and assimilation of food

VITAMIN B-COMPLEX — to avoid depletion from the system, helps build the body's resistance to disease and gives the body energy

VITAMIN C — protection for the whole system, protects the tissues to resist infections

VITAMIN D — helps calcium and minerals absorb, essential to maintain a normal basal metabolism

VITAMIN E — improves circulation and reduces uric acid, protects the body from virus

VITAMIN F — lubricant for cells giving tone and elasticity
CALCIUM — builds blood, assists digestive ferments and
    checks peristaltic action
MAGNESIUM — aids in prevention of constipation, alkalizes
    system
ZINC — aids digestion, assists body in absorbing B-complex
    vitamins
PURE WATER — cleans the bowels
FRESH FRUIT AND VEGETABLE JUICES — provide nut-
    rients easily assimilated
YOGURT — restores friendly bacteria in system
KEFIR — high in enzymes for healthy bowels
COMFREY AND PEPSIN — helps digest proteins
PAPAYA JUICE — aids digestion relieves infections in the
    colon and helps break down pus and mucus reached by the
    juice
BANANAS — valuable and soothing to bowels, must be ripe
MILLET — low in starch, easily digested
WHEY POWDER — high in nutrients, helps utilize calcium,
    easily digested
PROTEIN DIGESTIVE TABLETS — helps foods to digest and
    soothing to the bowels, important in helping to digest
    meat

ORTHODOX PRESCRIBED MEDICATION

SULFASALAZINE — it is used to help control inflammatory bowel disease such as enteritis or colitis

Common side effects:

Continuing headache	Itching
Increased sensitivity to	Rash
sunlight	

Less common:

Aching of joints and muscles	Unexplained sore throat or fever
Difficulty in swallowing	Unusual bleeding or bruising

Pale skin   Unusual tiredness or
Redness, blistering peeling or   weakness
   loosening of skin   Yellowing of eyes or skin

LUNGS

Mucus in the lungs is a chronic inflammatory disease of the lungs. It may result from croup, pneumonia, fibroid phthisis, fibrinous pleurisy, broncho-pneumonia, and irritations from inhaling air pollution.

Symptoms are cough, expectoration, and difficult breathing. Enemas have been helpful in cleaning poisons from the body to give it a chance to heal itself. Bronchitis is an infection in the bronchial tubes. Fever can occur. It is also accompanied by back and muscle pain, sore throat and a dry cough.

Asthma is a chronic respiratory condition characterized by difficulty in breathing, frequent coughing, and a feeling of suffocation. Attacks can be caused by emotional and physical stress, respiratory infection, air pollution or a change in the temperature.

The lungs are one of the elimination organs. Susceptibility to respiratory diseases are increased with air pollution, cigarette smoking, fatigue, chilling, malnutrition and allergic reactions.

HERBAL COMBINATIONS

No. 1 _____

COMFREY — healing for lungs, soothing and protective to the
      respiratory system
FENUGREEK — softens and dissolves hardened mucus, ex-
      pels phlegm and mucus, kills infections

No. 2

COMFREY—removes mucus, helps lower fevers and heals inflammation of tissues

MARSHMALLOW — heals and restores new cell tissues

MULLEIN — has antibiotic properties for upper respiratory system

SLIPPERY ELM — helps in inflammation of the mucus membranes, coats and soothes

LOBELIA — relaxes and clears the air passages of the lungs of viscid material

No. 3

COMFREY — removes mucus from the lungs, healing and soothing tonic

MARSHMALLOW — soothes irritated tissues of the lungs, removes difficult phlegm, relaxes the bronchial tubes

LOBELIA — removes obstructions from the respiratory system, relaxes and cleans the lungs

CHICKWEED — antiseptic to the blood, soothing to stomach and bowels, cleansing

MULLEIN — calming to irritated nerves, relieves pain, induces relaxed sleep, contains potassium and it is thought that the lack of potassium in the body which causes asthma

OTHER USES

ALLERGIES   HAY FEVER
ASTHMA   LUNG CONGESTION
BRONCHITIS   MUCUS
COUGHS   PNEUMONIA
CROUP   SINUS PROBLEMS
EMPHYSEMA   UPPER RESPIRATORY
                               SYSTEM

SPECIAL DIETARY HELPS

VITAMIN A — good for healing lung tissue
VITAMIN B-COMPLEX — (especially B12) builds the blood
VITAMIN B6 — deficiency occurs in some asthma patients
VITAMIN C — fights infection and speeds healing
VITAMIN D — works with vitamin A to help body withstand
    diseases
VITAMIN E — helps guard against air pollution, helps the
    body to use oxygen more efficiently in lung problems
BIOFLAVONOIDS WITH RUTIN — works with Vitamin C to
    strengthen capillaries
MULTI-VITAMIN AND MINERAL (NATURAL) — for
    overall body strength
FOLIC ACID — helps strengthen lungs
POTASSIUM — found in tomatoes, lettuce, turnips, dandelion
    greens, celery, egg plant, radishes, fresh string beans,
    brussel sprouts, kohlrabi, and mellons
BARLEY WATER — contains hordenine, which relieves
    bronchial spasms
DIET, CLEANSING — helps eliminate mucus; during a
    cleansing diet, germs are burned up or oxidized and elimi-
    nated and mucus is dispelled from the lungs
GARLIC—acts as an antibiotic in killing germs, helps dissolve
    mucus from the bronchial tubes, lungs and sinus passages
HONEY — cleans the lungs, soothes coughing spasms
JUICE, FRUIT FASTS — cleans and nourishes the body
JUICE, GRAPE — clears the mucus and phlegm from the lungs
VINEGAR AND WATER — has a cleansing effect
WATER, PURE — loss of fluids increases need
TEAS, HERBAL — cleans cells and provides nourishment
FRESH PINEAPPLE, BERRIES, most sour fruits help to dis-
    solve mucus from the lungs

ORTHODOX PRESCRIBED MEDICATION

PENICILLIN — antibiotics

Common side effects:

Hives	Rash
Itching	Wheezing

Less common side effects:

Diarrhea	Swelling of face and ankles
Nausea and vomiting	Unusual tiredness or weakness
Blood in the urine	Troubled breathing

TETRACYCLINE — for bronchitis and sore throat in children

Common side effects:

Ugly stain and deformity in developing teeth	Rash
Interferes with bone growth	Diarrhea
Stomach upset	Sore mouth

Widely used medication for Bronchial asthma are PREDNISONE and ISOPROTERENOL an inhalator.

Possible side effects:

Convulsions	Peptic ulcer
Glaucoma	Stunted growth in children

ISOPROTERENAL — abnormal heart rhythm and even death.

MENOPAUSE

Menopause is that period in a women's life which marks the permanent cessation of menstrual activity. It occurs between

35 to 58 years. Surgical menopause occurs in almost 30% of U.S. women aged 50-64. Menopausal symptoms are hot flashes, calcium disturbances, insomnia, diminished interest in sex, irritability, and instability. Poor diet, lack of exercise and emotional stress may increase the symptoms of menopause.

HERBAL COMBINATIONS

No. 1

BLACK COHOSH — contains natural estrogen, helps hot flashes, acts as a sedative to contract the uterus

LICORICE — stimulates adrenal glands, contains estrogen, supplies energy

FALSE UNICORN — stimulates reproductive organs, helps in uterine disorders, headaches and depression

SIBERIAN GINSENG — stimulates the entire body, nourishes the blood, corrects hormonal imbalance

SARSAPARILLA — contains progesterone and cortin to help achieve glandular balance

SQUAW VINE — uterine tonic, helps kidneys to eliminate urine

BLESSED THISTLE — good for menstrual disorders, headaches, tonic

OTHER USES

HORMONE IMBALANCE   MORNING SICKNESS
HOT FLASHES   SEXUAL IMPOTENCY
GLAND MALFUNCTIONING   UTERUS PROBLEMS
MENSTRUAL PROBLEMS

SPECIAL DIETARY HELPS

VITAMIN A — helps in maintaining normal glandular activity
VITAMIN B-COMPLEX — for nerves and iron absorption

VITAMIN B$_6$ — relieves swelling and water retention
VITAMIN C — helps build resistance to infection
RUTIN — helps in hemorrhoids, strengthens capillaries
VITAMIN E — increases production of hormones, promotes the functions of the sexual glands, helps relieve hot flashes and dryness in the vagina
VITAMIN F — promotes healing and builds tissues
MULTI VITAMIN AND MINERAL — natural, to give strength
PANTOTHENIC AND PABA — relieves nervous irritability
CALCIUM AND PHOSPHORUS BALANCE — bone meal, calcium can relieve hot flashes
IRON — for energy and oxygen
MAGNESIUM — works with B-complex to control the nerves
POTASSIUM — helps relieve swelling and muscle cramps
ACIDOPHILUS — can help in vaginitis and cystitis
BREWER'S YEAST — gives strength to the body, nourish the cells
GARLIC — can help in yeast infection
KELP — for anemia

ORTHODOX PRESCRIBED MEDICATION

ESTROGEN — hormone replacement

Common side effects are:

Blood clots	Shortness of breath
Breast, lumps	Cramps of lower stomach
Pains in chest, groins, and legs	Loss of appetite
	Nausea
Headache, severe, sudden	Swelling of ankles and feet
Speech, slurred, sudden	Swelling and increased
Loss of coordination	tenderness of breasts
Vision changes	

MIGRAINE HEADACHES

Migraine headaches are a type of headache due to the alternating constriction or dilation of the blood vessels in the brain. The exact cause is unknown, but emotional stress is thought to play a large role. The symptoms include intense pain, nausea, vomiting, and visual problems.

HERBAL COMBINATIONS

No. 1 _____

FENUGREEK — kills infection, strong antiseptic
THYME — antiseptic and healing powers, cleans stomach

OTHER USES

BRONCHITIS	HEARTBURN
DIGESTION	MUCUS
FEVERS	SINUS CONGESTION
HEADACHE	WORMS

SPECIAL DIETARY HELPS

VITAMIN B-COMPLEX — general nutrition, stimulant, utilizes energy in brain and nervous tissues
VITAMIN C — used daily will help protect from stress
CALCIUM — calms nerves, needed in stressful times
LECITHIN — helps control the nerves
MULTI-MINERAL — strengthen the system
NIACIN — prevents nervous disorders, promotes good physical and mental health
RUTIN — needed for healthy capillaries
WATER, PURE — cleans the system
BREWERS' YEAST — contains complete protein and B-complex, very helpful in migraine headaches

CARROT AND CELERY JUICE — said to relieve migraine headaches

SPROUTS — high in chlorophyll which is the life blood of plants, and is similar to human blood

VINEGAR — (apple cider) with honey in water has been said to relieve migraine headaches

Avoid red meats. They cause uric acid build up in system

ORTHODOX PRESCRIBED MEDICATION

INDERAL has become popular for migraine headaches. In older persons (over sixty), INDERAL seems to be eliminated from the body more slowly, so these people are more susceptible to side effects.

Possible side effects:

Tiredness	Stomach upset
Weakness	Diarrhea
Light-headedness	Breathing, (difficult)

METHYSERIDGE is claimed to cure migraine.

Side effects:

Ankles, swollen	Hair (falling out)
Cramps in calves of legs	Weight increase
Indigestion	

NERVOUS DISORDERS

Nervous disorders are manifested by the instability of nerve action, excitability, the state of restlessness, mental or physical or both. The nervous system is vital to life. The nervous system transmits all sensory input, sound, sight, taste, smell and touch to the brain and controls the workings of the organs. It helps maintain the temperature of the body and blood pressure. Causes of disorders can include lack of proper nutrition and organic disorders, overwork, worry, noisy surroundings and physical problems. Exercise, including breathing exercises (one nostril at a time), helps in nervous disorders.

HERBAL COMBINATIONS

No. 1 _____

BLACK COHOSH — contains alkaloid properties for nerves
CAPSICUM — stimulating to distribute other herbs to needed parts of the body
VALERIAN — pain reliever, relaxing for nervous tension
MISTLETOE — tones and strengthens the nerves, natural tranquilizer
GINGER — helps hold together all herbs, helps relaxant herbs work more effectively
ST. JOHNSWORT — excellent for pain
HOPS — its sedative properties make an excellent relaxant, contains B vitamins for nerves
WOOD BETONY — nervine helps in hysteria, useful when used with other herbs

No. 2 _____

BLACK COHOSH — soothing effect on the nervous system, lowers blood pressure
CAPSICUM — stimulates other herbs to be more effective, increases blood circulation, helps eliminates toxic wastes
VALERIAN — sedative effect on the entire system, remedy for nervous disorders
MISTLETOE — gives tone to the nerves, re-establishes circulation of the blood
LADY'S SLIPPER — tonic for exhausted nervous system, calming to body and mind

LOBELIA — powerful relaxant on the nerves, healing powers to the blood vessels

SCULLCAP — controls nervous irritations, good for insomnia due to overactive mind

HOPS — general tonic, sleep inducer, sedative to the nervous system

WOOD BETONY — cleans impurities from blood, effective sedative

OTHER USES

ANXIETY	INSOMNIA
CONVULSIONS	NERVOUS BREAKDOWN
HEADACHES	RELAXANT
HYPERACTIVITY	STRESS
HYSTERIA	

SPECIAL DIETARY HELPS

VITAMIN A — works with vitamins D and E to fight infections and promote growth repair of body tissues.

B VITAMINS — necessary for normal functioning of the nervous system

B_1 — important to a healthy nervous system and effects mental attitude

B_3 — helps depression

B_{12} — necessary for healthy nerves and brain, prevents nervous disorders

B_6 — soothing effect on nerves, prevents nervous disorders

VITAMIN C — works with vitamin D in the regulation of calcium metabolism, promotes health in the system, lack of vitamin C causes irritability

CALCIUM — relaxing and calming to the nerves, manganese is necessary for proper absorption

VITAMIN D — also a nerve vitamin, helps to relax

IRON — promotes a sense of well-being, increases energy and vitality

LYSINE (AMINO ACID) — lack causes irritability

MAGNESIUM — feeds the nerves, helps emotional disturbances

NIACIN — produces happy feelings

PANTOTHENIC ACID — strengthens to withstand stress

POTASSIUM — strengthens the nervous system

TYROSINE (AMINO ACID) — controls depression, along with B_6 and niacin

APPLES — health tonic and regulates the bowels, apples are said to prevent emotional upsets, tension and headaches

ARTICHOKES — cleans the kidneys, helps with poor digestion

BLACKSTRAP MOLASSES (UNSULPHURED) — rich in iron, gives the body energy

BRAN — contains natural amino acids, necessary for healthy body, keeps the colon clean

BREWER'S YEAST — supplies live protein and B vitamins

BRUSSELS SPROUTS — tonic food, good for catarrh build-up

CAULIFLOWER — purifies the blood, rich in minerals

FRUIT — papaya, guava, acerola, gives nourishment to the body, aids digestion, cleans the digestive tract

LETTUCE — calming to the nerves

TEAS — Fenugreek, Chamomile (has a tranquilizing effect), also cleans the system of impurities

VEGETABLES, RAW JUICES — carrot, beet and cabbage, cleansing and nourishing to the body

WHEAT GERM — excellent source of the B-complex vitamins

WHOLE GRAINS — buckwheat, barley, millet

ORTHODOX PRESCRIBED MEDICATION

VALIUM — is prescribed for nervous tension.

Common side effects:

Clumsiness	Dizziness
Unsteadiness	Drowsiness

Less common side effects:

Blurred vision	Withdrawal symptoms
Constipation	Nausea
Diarrhea	Slurred speech
Headache	Stomach pains
Heartburn	Unusual tiredness

PANCREAS

The Pancreas gland performs two important functions. It is necessary to produce the pancreatic acid juice which is used to help digestion, and it also produces insulin.

Pancreatitis symptoms can be acid indigestion, nausea, pain and gas.

HERBAL COMBINATIONS

No. 1 _____

GOLDEN SEAL — natural insulin, regulates sugar in the blood, feeds glands, builds resistance to diseases

JUNIPER BERRIES — high in natural insulin, helps restore function of the pancreas

UVA URSI — helps regulate sugar levels, helps alleviate pancreas disorders

HUCKLEBERRY — high in natural insulin, helps alleviate hyperglycemia

MULLEIN — antibiotic properties, nourishes body strength, calms nerves

COMFREY — soothing and healing to all parts of the body, high in protein, nutritious

YARROW — blood cleanser, dilates the pores, producing sweating, removes congestion

GARLIC — stimulates cell growth and activity, rejuvenates

body functions

CAPSICUM — helps heal pancreas, increases and regulates circulation, nourishes

DANDELION — increases activity of the pancreas, clears obstructions, purifies the blood, tonic

MARSHMALLOW — healing to the system, removes phlegm, high in vitamin A and minerals

BUCHU — beneficial to eliminate excess uric acid, healing to genito-urinary tract

BISTORT — beneficial for infectious disease, tonic to body, contains some insulin

LICORICE — increases strength of other herbs, supplies energy to system

No. 2 _____

JUNIPER — high in natural insulin, helps restore function of pancreas, natural antibiotic

UVA URSI — helps regulate excess sugar in system, helps alleviate pancreas disorders

LICORICE — supplies energy to system, increases strength of other herbs

CAPSICUM — healing effect on the pancreas, increases and regulates circulation

MULLEIN — calming effect to the nerves, nourishes and strengthens the body, antibiotic

GOLDEN SEAL — natural insulin, regulates sugar levels, strengthens glands to build resistance to diseases, builds natural immunity

OTHER USES

BLOOD SUGAR PROBLEMS	GLYCOSURIA
GALL BLADDER	KIDNEY
FASTING HYPERGLYCEMIA	LIVER
GLUCOSE INTOLERANCE	SPLEEN

SPECIAL DIETARY HELPS

VITAMIN A — assists in maintaining normal glandular activity
VITAMIN B-COMPLEX — general nutritional stimulant
VITAMIN C — promotes glandular activity, helps infections
VITAMIN E — reduces uric acid, increases production of hormones
CALCIUM — calms nerves, builds blood, promotes enzyme stimulation
MAGNESIUM — stimulates the glands, alkalizes the system
MANGANESE — essential element, acts as an activator for enzymes
NIACIN — promotes growth by stimulating metabolic processes
POTASSIUM — increases glandular secretions
ZINC — aids entire hormonal system and all the glands
FRUITS, RAW, FRESH — cleans the intestines, nourishes
MOLASSES — rich in iron
NUTS — contains protein needed for cells
SE_DS, PUMPKIN — cleansing and nourishing to the body, helps carry nourishment to various parts of the body
VEGETABLES, GREEN LEAFY — supplies live enzymes
RAW FOOD — stimulates the pancreas to increase insulin production
PROTEIN — (such as cottage cheese, yogurt, kefir, nuts and seeds, and avocado), is necessary for all the cells of the body

ORTHODOX PRESCRIBED MEDICATION

INSULIN — insulin belongs to the group of medicines called hormones. If the body does not make enough insulin to meet its needs, a condition known as diabetes mellitus (sugar diabetes) may develop. Eating the right foods along with proper exercise plus insulin helps keep health in balance.

Insulin is made from beef or pork sources, and many insulin preparations contain mixtures of both. Insulin must be injected under the skin, because when taken by mouth, it is destroyed by stomach acid.

Insulin reaction may occur and the symptoms are:

Anxiety	Headache
Chills	Nausea
Cold sweats	Nervousness
Cool pale skin	Rapid pulse
Drowsiness	Shakiness
Excessive hunger	Unusual tiredness or weakness

PARASITES

A parasite is an organism that lives within, upon, or at the expense of another organism, known as the host, without contributing ɔ the survival of the host. Parasites are said to affect a large percentage of our population, causing many symptoms often blamed on other conditions such as pneumonia, jaundice or periodontitis. Symptoms can include diarrhea, hunger pain, appetite loss, weight loss and anemia. Tape worms can be contracted from eating insufficiently cooked meats, especially beef, pork, and fish.

HERBAL COMBINATIONS

No. 1 _____

PUMPKIN SEEDS — expels tapeworms efficiently, nutritious
CULVERS ROOT — promotes intestinal secretions, tonic and
    gentle to the liver
MANDRAKE — contains anti-tumor compounds, glandular
    stimulant, liver cleanser

VIOLET — contains properties that will reach places only the
blood and lymphatic fluids penetrate
COMFREY — excellent body cleanser, over-all tonic, heals
and nourishes the system
CASCARA SAGRADA — safe laxative and cleanser, stimulating effect on the colon
WITCH HAZEL — useful for internal inflamed conditions,
stops internal bleeding
MULLEIN — calming effect on all inflamed and irritated
nerves, good for bleeding bowels
SLIPPERY ELM — soothes and disperses inflammation, draws
out impurities, heals all parts of the body

OTHER USES

BOWEL (CLEANS)	TUMORS
CANCER	TOXINS (REMOVES)
PROSTATE	WORMS

SPECIAL DIETARY HELPS

VITAMIN A — improves resistance to infections in the gastro-
intestinal tract
VITAMIN B-COMPLEX — builds blood, tones muscles, acts
as a general nutrition stimulant
VITAMIN B_6 — promotes appetite, digestion, assimilation and
elimination
VITAMIN B_{12} — improves blood supply, promotes growth,
prevents nervous disorders
VITAMIN C — detoxifies the body and strengthens the body
VITAMIN D — necessary for good body form and health
VITAMIN K — aids in blood coagulation and controls consis-
tency
CALCIUM — promotes enzyme stimulation, calms nerves,
used as a pain killer
IRON — increases energy and vitality, alkalizes the system

FRUITS, FRESH, RAW — promotes healthy body with live
  enzymes
GARLIC — antibiotic, helps destroy parasites
VEGETABLES, FRESH, RAW — promotes healthy body
  with live enzymes
A clean colon will help eliminate the breeding place for parasites. Whole wheat bread, instead of white; honey, instead
  of white sugar; natural vitamins and minerals, instead of
  those made in a laboratory, should be used.

ORTHODOX PRESCRIBED MEDICATION

Some medicines are effective, but can be a shock to the
system and can inhibit the function of the liver and other organs.
PYRVINIUM — POVAN — used for pinworm infesta-
tions. This medicine is a dye and will cause the stools to be red.
It may also stain the teeth.

Possible side effects:

Nausea   Dizziness
Vomiting — may occur and   Unusual sensitivity of skin
  will be red in color   to sunlight
Skin rash   Stomach cramps
Diarrhea

PAIN

A disturbed sensation where a person suffers discomfort or
distress due to provocation of sensory nerves. Pain is a
symptom, and the reason for the pain is the important thing to
seek. There could be many reasons for pain in the system. It
could cause emotional stress with lack of sleep. Therefore, it is
important to find a natural relief for pain.

HERBAL COMBINATIONS

No. 1 _____ _____

VALERIAN — nerve tonic, relieves headache pain
WILD LETTUCE — helps after-birth pains, general pain re-
    liever
CAPSICUM — stimulant, relaxant

OTHER USES

AFTER-BIRTH PAIN	RELAXANT
CRAMPS	TOOTHACHE
HEADACHE	

SPECIAL DIETARY HELPS

VITAMIN B-COMPLEX — especially B_1, B_2, B_6, and B_{12},
    calming to the nerves
VITAMIN A — lubricates all membranes to help keep them
    clean and free from virus infections
VITAMIN C — detoxifies germs in body
VITAMIN D — relaxes nerves and helps calcium to absorb
VITAMIN E — dilates capillary blood vessels to lessen pain
CALCIUM — helps in menstrual pain, calms nerves
FOLIC ACID — needed under stress and disease
MAGNESIUM — helps the nervous system, it promotes sleep
PANTOTHENIC ACID — helps the body to withstand stress
FRUIT, JUICES — assimilates quickly into the blood stream
VEGETABLES, FRESH, JUICES — cleans and nourishes the
    body
WILD YAM — has been used for many kinds of pain

ORTHODOX PRESCRIBED MEDICATION

    ASPIRIN and related products.

Possible side effects:

Stomach irritation   Ringing in the ears
Brain hemorrhage   Nausea
Birth defects   Bleeding stomach
Arteriosclerosis   Allergic reaction
Destroys vitamin C and others

Could possibly cause ulcers and be dangerous to ulcer patients.

POTASSIUM

Potassium can be considered generally as the mineral foundation of the muscular tissues, assuring their elasticity. Potassium and sodium help regulate the water balance within the body. It also helps to normalize the heartbeat and nourish the muscular system. It is necessary for normal growth, and is important to preserve proper alkalinity of body fluids. It also stimulates nerve impulses for muscle contraction, as well as the kidneys to eliminate poisonous body wastes. Potassium assists in the conversion of glucose to glycogen, the form in which glucose can be stored in the liver.

HERBAL COMBINATIONS

No. 1 _____

KELP — minerals and trace elements are strengthening to the
        system, strengthens the blood
DULSE — high in minerals, promotes glandular health,
        strengthens tissues of the heart and brain
WATERCRESS — rich in vitamins and minerals, enriches the
        blood, increases physical endurance

WILD CABBAGE — contains silica, iron and maganese, calming to the system

HORSERADISH — stimulating for metabolism, contains sulphur, potassium, and is rich in vitamin C. It is an antispasmodic herb.

HORSETAIL — diaphoretic, rich in silica which aids the circulation contains calcium, iron, phosphorus, rich in minerals; improves skin tones

OTHER USES

ALLERGIES	FEVER
CONGESTIVE HEART FAILURE	FRACTURES
CONSTIPATION	HYPERTENSION
COLIC	SEVERE INJURIES
DIARRHEA	SUCH AS BURNS
INSOMNIA	

SPECIAL DIETARY HELPS

BANANA — dried—rich in potassium, helps prevent germs from accumulating in tissues

JUICE, RAW POTATO — rich in potassium for the adrenal glands

MINT LEAVES — rich in potassium

POTATOES — baked—the skin is rich in potassium, fresh— contains moderate amounts of potassium

SEEDS, SUNFLOWER — rich in potassium and protein

VEGETABLES, GREEN, LEAFY — high in minerals

WHOLE GRAINS — rice bran especially is rich in potassium

ORTHODOX PRESCRIBED MEDICATION

ASPIRIN and other medications cause a loss of potassium in the urine.

Soft drink: too much can cause loss of potassium.

THIAZIDE DIURETICS — a medicine that is prescribed

to help reduce the amount of water in the body by increasing the flow of urine.

The loss of potassium is increased when using diuretics.

PRENATAL

There are a lot of changes in a pregnant woman, both mental and physical. The blood supply increases, there can be nausea, and the need for sleep increases. The Nutritional needs of the mother increase, and the condition of the child as well as the mother could be improved by dietary supplementation.

One way to prepare for the delivery of the child is with the use of herbs. They have been found to help strengthen the uterus for safe and easy delivery.

HERBAL COMBINATIONS

No. 1 _____

BLACK COHOSH — controls hemorrhaging, nervousness and delivery pains; reduces high blood pressure
SQUAW VINE — useful for urinary and vaginal infections, helps facilitate delivery, strengthens uterus in childbirth
LOBELIA — sedative for nerves, eliminates congestion
PENNYROYAL — mild, tranquil effect on central nervous system, helpful for safe delivery
RED RASPBERRY — strengthens uterus, relieves pain, aids in easy labor

No. 2 _____

BLACK COHOSH — helps in uterine disorders, works as sedative for headaches, lowers blood pressure

FALSE UNICORN — tonic for system, strengthens the ovaries, rich in trace minerals

SQUAW VINE — works as a natural sedative on the nerves, stimulates and regulates the amount of contractions

BLESSED THISTLE — helps promote natural flow of breast milk, eliminates mucus congestion

LOBELIA — mild sedative, useful in urinary problems, eliminates congestion

PENNYROYAL — useful just before delivery, works on the central nervous system

RED RASPBERRY — strengthens female organs, prevents hemorrhaging and regulates muscle contractions in the uterus during delivery and reduces false labor pains

OTHER USES

CHILD BIRTH   DELIVERY
MENSTRUAL CRAMPS   HORMONE REGULATOR
UTERUS (STRENGTHENS)

SPECIAL DIETARY HELPS

VITAMIN B-COMPLEX — especially B_6, soothes the nerves, increases relaxation, restores sleep, prevents morning sickness and nausea in pregnancy

VITAMIN C — kills infections, promotes formation of healthy teeth, strengthens blood vessels, builds resistance to infections

VITAMIN D — regulates mineral metabolism of bones, teeth and nails

VITAMIN K — to help blood coagulation and to prevent hemorrhages in delivery

BIOFLAVONOIDS — to strengthen blood vessels

CALCIUM — high amounts needed for bones teeth (baby utilizes high amounts)

IRON — enriches blood, feeds tissues, nourishes the glands

THIAMINE — in late pregnancy, builds the blood, tones muscles, nutritional stimulant, feeds nerves
FRUITS, FRESH — gives strength and nourishment to the body
PROTEIN — gives daily nourishment of the cells (milk, yogurt, whole-grains, nuts, beans, lentils, eggs, cheese and fish)
VEGETABLES, FRESH — gives necessary vitamins and minerals to the body

ORTHODOX PRESCRIBED MEDICATION

Avoid caffeinated drinks, stay away from antacids, baking soda as sodium will increase fluid retention.
Birth defects could be a result of fetus-damaging drugs, bacterial infections, poor nutrition and viral infections.

PROSTATE

Prostatitis is an inflammation of the male sex gland, the prostate. Herbs can play an important role to a healthy prostate, bladder and kidney function. It can help in keeping these free from infection. Herbs help in the relief of chronic irritations of the bladder. Eating correct food and getting sufficient exercise in the fresh air also helps.

HERBAL COMBINATIONS

No. 1 _____

BLACK COHOSH — stimulates secretions of the liver, kidneys and lymph glands, expels mucus
LICORICE — removes excess fluid from the body, supplies

energy, acts as a natural cortisone

KELP — promotes glandular health, relieves inflammation and reduces pain in glands

GOTU KOLA — natural diuretic, defends body against toxins, helps with hormone balance

GOLDEN SEAL — antibiotic and antiseptic to stop infection, eliminates toxins from bladder

CAPSICUM — stimulating, reduces glandular swellings, distributes other herbs

GINGER — helps remove excess waste from system, enhances effectiveness of other herbs, stimulates

LOBELIA — removes obstructions from any part of the body, relaxant and stimulant

No. 2

JUNIPER BERRIES — high in vitamin C and other antiseptic properties

GOLDEN SEAL — relieves painful inflammation, strong antibiotic and antiseptic properties

CAPSICUM — stimulates all herbs to needed parts, helps reduce swellings

PARSLEY — work to stop infection and inflammation in prostate, high in vitamin A, B, and iron

GINGER — aids in holding herbs together, kills parasites in prostate

SIBERIAN GINSENG — strengthens the system

UVA URSI — antiseptic properties to clear infection

MARSHMALLOW — helps the body build new tissues, heals sores

QUEEN OF THE MEADOW — natural diuretic

OTHER USES

BLADDER	LIVER
HORMONE REGULATOR	SPLEEN
KIDNEYS	URINARY TRACT

SPECIAL DIETARY HELPS

VITAMIN A — helps in tension, irritability; helps infections
VITAMIN B-COMPLEX — especially B6, helps in hormone
    balance
VITAMIN C — helps resist infection
VITAMIN E — essential for reproduction, stimulates male
    hormone
VITAMIN F — aids in prostate gland problems
ZINC — helps absorb B vitamin stimulates prostate
CALCIUM — helps minerals to absorb
MAGNESIUM — necessary for calcium and vitamin C
    metabolism
ALMONDS AND SESAME SEEDS — high in calcium and
    potassium, valuable for nourishing the cells
ARTICHOKES — cleanses the prostate and urinary tract
ASPARAGUS — natural diuretic
BEE POLLEN — stimulates male potency, heals prostate trou-
    bles
GRAINS — contains quality proteins and the B-complex vita-
    min
PUMPKIN SEEDS — healing and nourishing to the prostate
    and urinary tract
RAW FRUITS AND VEGETABLES — provides enzymes
    necessary for healthy system
SUNFLOWER SEEDS — high in protein and enzymes
WATER — drink lots of pure water to clean the system
WATERCRESS, PARSLEY — natural diuretic

ORTHODOX PRESCRIBED MEDICATION

NALIDIXIC ACID — for prostate infection.

Common side effects:

Blurred or decreased vision	Diarrhea
Double vision	Itching
Change in color vision	Nausea

Over-brightness of lights
Halos around lights

Rash
Vomiting

Rare side effects:

Dizziness
Drowsiness
Dark urine
Pale skin
Pale stools
Severe stomach pain

Unusual bleeding
Unexplained sore throat
   or fever
Unusual tiredness or weakness
Yellowing of eyes or skin

REDUCING AID

Losing weight is a matter of curbing the amount of food calories eaten, and increasing daily activities. There is no easy road to reducing. The American public should stop hoping for an easy way to lose weight. The only hope is to stop believing that there is one, and start changing to thin eating habits. It has taken years to accumulate excess weight and it will take months to lose.

Herbs can help the body adjust as well as supply vitamins and minerals. This combination acts as a general body cleanser, regulates metabolism, dissolves fat in the body, helps eliminate craving for food, stimulates glandular secretions, reduces water retention, boosts energy and helps in constipation.

HERBAL COMBINATIONS

No. 1 _____

CHICKWEED — dissolves fat in blood vessels, potassium
      content helps eliminate craving for food
MANDRAKE — cleans liver, eliminates constipation, stimu-
      lates glands

LICORICE — gives energy boost, counteracts stress, helps balance other herbs

SAFFLOWER — helps produce more adrenalin, natural insulin, digestive aid

ECHINACEA — purifies blood for good feeling, lymphatic cleanser, helps in weight loss

BLACK WALNUT — balances sugar levels, burns excess toxins and fatty materials

GOTU KOLA — feeds the brain, energizes cells of the brain, gives strength

HAWTHORNE — strengthens heart, helps circulation, good for nerves and stress

PAPAYA — calms nervous stomach, and aids digestion

FENNEL — cleans mucous membranes of intestinal tract, and removes waste from body

DANDELION — strengthens liver, helps in water retention and destroys acids

OTHER USES

ENERGY   CLEANSER
CONSTIPATION   WATER RETENTION

SPECIAL DIETARY HELPS

VITAMIN B-COMPLEX — especially B_6 and B_{12}, necessary for normal metabolism of nerve tissue and is involved in protein, fat and carbohydrate metabolism

VITAMIN C — increases alertness, promotes health

VITAMIN E — promotes circulation, reduces uric acid

VITAMIN F — improves heart action

PHENYLALANINE (NATURAL AMINO ACID) — has an effect on the thyroid to help weight control, depresses the appetite

CALCIUM — calms the nerves, promotes sleep, builds the blood, assists

LECITHIN — helps break up the fatty material in body, distributes body weight, maintains healthy nervous system.

MAGNESIUM — stimulate the glands, creates good disposition

PROTEIN (VEGETABLE) — such as in grains, seeds and nuts

BREWER'S YEAST — strengthens the body and gives energy

KELP — helps regulate thyroid for metabolism

PINEAPPLE — aid to digestion to help rid the body of excess weight

WATERCRESS — rich in minerals and vitamins and chlorophyll

WHEAT GERM — contains vitamin B-complex protein

ALL HEALTH BUILDING FOODS — cut the amount you usually eat and cut out sweets

ORTHODOX PRESCRIBED MEDICATION

DEXEDRINE — it is usually prescribed for short-term adjunct to caloric restriction. Could be habit-forming, hypertension.

Common side effects:

False sense of well-being	Restlessness
Irritability	Trouble in sleeping
Nervousness	

CAUTION: After such stimulant effects have worn off, drowsiness, trembling, unusual tiredness or weakness, or mental depression may occur.

SEX REJUVENATION

This combination has been used for male hormone problems such as impotence. The main impact on the male hormone testosterone is on the emotions. If production were to cease, it would produce irritable, fretful, and sleepless feelings. Memory would begin to fail, and some men feel the hot flashes that women often have at menopause.

HERBAL COMBINATIONS

No. 1

SIBERIAN GINSENG — antistress, benefits heart and circulation, stimulates body energy, contains male hormone, testosterone, helps correct impotence

ECHINACEA — excellent blood purifier, increases body's resistance to infection, good for enlargement and weakness of the prostate gland

SAW PALMETTO — effective hormone herb useful on reproductive glands, tonic to system, it is said to increase the size of small breasts

GOTU KOLA — rebuilds energy reserve, helps in nervous disorders, strengthens heart, brain and nerves, helps with hormone balance

DAMIANA — helps balance female hormones, hot flashes, stimulating to the system, increases sperm count in the male and strengthens the egg in the female, helps in sexual impotence

SARSAPARILLA — contains progesterone for glandular balance, stimulates circulation, contains male hormone, testosterone

PERIWINKLE — carries oxygen to the brain, nourishes and stimulates the system

GARLIC — natural antibiotic, reduces blood pressure, stimulates cell growth

CAPSICUM — stimulates other herbs to the location where they are needed, wards off disease, increases blood circulation

CHICKWEED — dissolves plaque out of blood vessels, contains antiseptic properties

OTHER USES

FRIGIDITY   SEXUAL STIMULANT
HOT FLASHES   STERILITY
MENOPAUSE

SPECIAL DIETARY HELPS

VITAMIN A — lessens pre-menstrual tension and irritability
VITAMIN B-COMPLEX — especially B₆, helps in hormonal
  and sugar balance
VITAMIN C AND BIOFLAVONOIDS — increases capillary
  strength
VITAMIN D — relaxes nerves
VITAMIN E — male hormone energizer which helps build up
  the male sex glands for youthful hormone balance
VITAMIN F — alieviates female problems
CALCIUM AND MAGNESIUM — helps correct hormone
  rhythm, nerve foods
DOLOMITE AND BONE MEAL — contains calcium so
  necessary for over-all healthy feeling
IRON — enriches blood
MANGANESE
PANTOTHENIC ACID AND PABA — relieves nervous ir
  ritability
ZINC — stimulates prostate glands
FRESH FRUIT (TREE RIPENED)
PROTEIN (NOT RED MEAT) — grains, nuts and seeds, wheat
  germ, polished rice
SEEDS, SUNFLOWER AND PUMPKIN — stimulates male
  potency and heals prostate problems
TEA, FENUGREEK — soothing on the urinary tract, keeping it
  free from mucus and pus
TEA, PARSLEY — relieves bladder irritations, high in vitamin
  A, has a healing and moisturizing effect on mucous lining

of prostate gland
VEGETABLES, FRESH — live enzymes, nourishment

ORTHODOX PRESCRIBED MEDICATION

ANDROID — prescribed for impotence

Possible side effects:

Skin rash
Shock
Deficient sperm count

Gynecomastia & abnormal mammary glands in male, could secrete milk)

SKIN

The skin is the largest eliminative organ of the body. If it is functioning properly, it eliminates on a par with the kidneys and the lungs. Sun and fresh air are important to the skin. Olive Oil or Aloe Vera are good for sun bathing, for they do not plug the pores. The use of Loftah or Sponge is useful when bathing to stimulate and tone the skin and remove dead skin from the body.

HERBAL COMBINATIONS

No. 1 _____

DULSE — high in iodine, high in minerals and vitamins needed for the skin, hair and nails
HORSETAIL — helps prevent falling hair and strengthens nails and tones the skin, high in minerals
SAGE — stimulates hair growth, an astringent and acts as a scalp tonic
ROSEMARY — strengthens eye sight, stimulates the skin and strengthens the hair

OTHER USES

HAIR   NAILS

SPECIAL DIETARY HELPS

VITAMIN A — promotes healthy skin
VITAMIN B-COMPLEX — especially B₂ (promotes healthier
    skin) and B₆ (helps prevent acne)
VITAMIN D — necessary for good body form
VITAMIN E — good for liver spots
CALCIUM — promotes skin healing
ZINC — helps in tissue respiration
BLACKSTRAP MOLASSES — provides iron for rich blood
BREWER'S YEAST — contains protein and B vitamins
DIET — a cleansing diet is beneficial for cleaning the blood to
    promote healthy skin
FRUITS, FRESH, RAW — cleans the blood to help keep the
    skin clear and healthy looking
GARLIC — the oil heals blisters, boils can be helped with oil
    and garlic, kills staphylococci germs in boils, heals run-
    ning sores
GRAINS, WHOLE — brown rice and millet, gives the body
    necessary protein for healthy skin
HONEY — good for sting bites
LECITHIN — helps in the structural support of all cells, espe-
    cially the nerves and brain
LEMON JUICE — helps skin conditions
SPROUTS — promotes healthy skin with enzyme, vitamins
    and mineral content
SEEDS, SUNFLOWER — protein, natural food, nourishes the
    entire body, helps dry skin
VEGETABLES, FRESH, RAW — nourishes the blood for
    healthy skin and body
WHEAT GERM OIL — good on sting bites
Avoid excess fat and sweets and any products with white flour
    and sugar

ORTHODOX PRESCRIBED MEDICATION

CLINDAMYCIN — CLEOCINT — external use — (Precautions) Mild stinging or burning may be expected. May cause the skin to become unusually dry. Do not get this medicine in the eyes or on the mouth or lips.

Possible side effects:

Chapped skin   Mild diarrhea
Itching, rash, redness, swelling

Rare, but possible side effects:

Severe stomach cramps   Severe, watery diarrhea, which
Pain   may be accompanied by
Bloating   blood mucus, and pus

THYROID

The chief function of the thyroid gland is to regulate the rate of metabolism. Goiter may be caused by a lack of iodine in the diet, inflammation of the thyroid gland due to infection or under or over production of hormones by the thyroid gland.

HERBAL COMBINATIONS

No. 1 _____

IRISH MOSS — purifies and strengthens the cellular structure and vital fluids of the system
KELP — promotes glandular health, highest natural source of iodine, rich in minerals, strengthens tissues in the brain and heart

BLACK WALNUT — helps to balance sugar levels, natural source of iodine, burns up excess toxins
PARSLEY — increases resistance to infection and diseases, high in potassium, regulates the fluids, tonic to urinary system
WATERCRESS — acts as a tonic for regulating metabolism, blood purifier
SARSAPARILLA — stimulates the metabolic rate, valuable in glandular balance
ICELAND MOSS — nutrient, tonic, regulates gastric acid

No. 2

KELP — promotes glandular health, helps control metabolism, high in minerals, cleans colon
IRISH MOSS — purifies and strengthens cellular structure, iodine helps glandular system
PARSLEY — tonic effect to the whole system, increases resistance to disease, high in minerals for healthy metabolism
CAPSICUM — stimulates blood circulation, helps other herbs to be more effective

OTHER USES

ENERGY	GOITER
EPILEPSY	HORMONES
FATIGUE	LYMPHATIC SYSTEM
GLANDS	

SPECIAL DIETARY HELPS

VITAMIN A — assists in sustaining normal glandular activity
VITAMIN B-COMPLEX — prime source of pre-digested protein, boosts the thyroid for energy
VITAMIN B6 — protects against stress, aids in formation of antibodies

VITAMIN C — neutralizes infections, helps promote healthy glandular function

VITAMIN E — increases production of hormones, improves circulation

CALCIUM — assists all metabolic functions to perform efficiently, promotes enzyme stimulation

IODINE — aids in the development and functioning of the thyroid gland and produces the hormone thyroxine, regulates the body's production of energy

ZINC — boosts the thyroid for energy

BREWER'S YEAST — contains nucleic acids and oil

EGGS, RAW, FERTILE — rich in protein, contains all the amino acids to combine with enzymes to build strong bodies

EXERCISE — daily exercise to circulate the blood which helps the thyroid

FRUIT, RAW, FRESH — easily assimilated enzyme that contains pre-digested levulose. The system instantly absorbs levulose to give the body energy and vigor.

SEEDS, PUMPKIN — contains protein, unsaturated fatty acids and minerals which unite with enzymes for a healthy hormonal function

SEEDS SUNFLOWER — high in proteins and vitamins and minerals, packed full of the sun

SPROUTS — live enzymes, easily assimilated, high in vitamins and amino acids, rich in chlorophyll, similar to human blood

YOGURT — richest source of enzymes, helps in assimilation of calcium, aids in the manufacture of B-complex, prime source of predigested protein

ORTHODOX PRESCRIBED MEDICATION

METHIMAZOLE — Antithyroid agents. They are used to treat conditions in which the thyroid gland produces too much thyroid hormone and also before thyroid surgery.

Possible side effects:

Itching	Numbness
Dizziness	Tingling of fingers
Joint pain	Skin rash
Loss of taste	Stomach pain
Nausea and vomiting	

ULCERS

Ulcers are open sores or lesions of the skin or mucous membranes of the body, with loss of substance, sometimes accompanied by formation of pus. Some nutritionists call stomach and gastric ulcers a deficiency disease caused by unhealthy tissue as a result of eating incompatible combinations of food leaving fermentation and putrefaction as the end-product.

Severe nervous and mental stress can cause ulcers. It is important to be able to relax and rest and free the mind of problems and stressful situations.

HERBAL COMBINATIONS

No. 1 _____

CAPSICUM — stimulant, hemorrhages, internal disinfectant, high in vitamins and minerals

GOLDEN SEAL — stops infection, internal bleeding, eliminates toxins from the stomach

MYRRH GUM — antiseptic, strengthens digestive system, aids inflammation to speed healing

OTHER USES

BAD BREATH   DYSENTERY
CANKER SORES   HEARTBURN
COLITIS   INDIGESTION
COLON   STOMACH ULCER
DIVERTICULITIS

SPECIAL DIETARY HELPS

VITAMIN A — large amounts at first complaint heals tissues
      that line the sores
VITAMIN B-COMPLEX — especially B$_2$ and B$_{12}$, improves
      the body health and strengthens the nerves
VITAMIN C AND BIOFLAVONOIDS — large amounts will
      help heal ulcers
VITAMINS E AND A TOGETHER — vitamin E helps heal
      scar tissue
VITAMIN K — helps in blood clotting
IRON — builds rich blood, gives energy to the body
BUTTERMILK — soothes the stomach
CABBAGE JUICE — heals ulcers
CHLOROPHYLL — liquid is good to take in water for cleaning
      the blood
COMFREY TEA — very healing, nourishing
RAW CABBAGE AND POTATO JUICE — contains vitamin
      P which helps ulcers heal
YOGURT — friendly stomach bacteria, prime source of pre-
      digested protein
Eliminate white sugar products and red meat

ORTHODOX PRESCRIBED MEDICATION

      CIMETIDINE (TAGAMET) — prescribed in treating cer-
tain types of ulcers

Common side effects:

Dizziness	Skin rash
Diarrhea	Swelling of breasts
Headaches	Breast soreness
Muscle Cramps	

Cleasing Diet

A cleansing diet is good during colds, flu or illness. The body has the ability to rid itself of toxins if it is given the chance. Toxins are expelled through the skin, which needs to be kept clean and scrubbed, and through the nose, mouth, colon and stomach. The purpose of cleansing the body is to eliminate excessive mucus and toxins. The first step is to stay away from white sugar products, white flour products, animal protein and salt.

My favorite cleansing diet is the No. 1 by Stanley Burrough. I sometimes use it for one day or as long as a week.

The benefits of a cleansing fast is it dissolves toxins and mucus in the body. It cleanses the kidneys and the digestive system. It purifies the glands and the cells. It eliminates build-up waste and hardened material in the joints and muscles. It relieves the pressure and irritation in the nerves, arteries and blood vessels. It builds a healthy bloodstream and increases spiritual awareness.

The lemon used in this diet is a loosening and cleansing agent with many important building factors. The ability of the elements in the lemon and the maple syrup along with the cayenne pepper work together to create the following results:

Potassium content strengthens and energizes the heart, stimulates and builds the kidneys and adrenal glands.

Oxygen content builds vitality.

Carbon acts as a motor stimulant.

Hydrogen activates the sensory nervous system.

Calcium strengthens and builds the lungs.

Phosphorus knits the bones, stimulates and builds the brain for clearer thinking.

Sodium encourages tissue building.

Magnesium acts as a blood alkalizer.

Iron builds the red corpuscles to rapidly correct the most common forms of anemia.

Chlorine cleanses the blood plasma.

Silicon aids the thyroid for deeper breathing.

The natural iron, copper, calcium, carbon, and hydrogen found in the sweetening supplies more building and cleansing material.

The cayenne pepper is necessary as it breaks up mucus and increases warmth by building the blood for an additional lift. It also adds many of the B vitamins and vitamin C.

Cleansing Diet No. 1

Master Cleanser by Stanley Burroughs
A method of cleaning without enemas

    2 Tbsp. fresh lemon or lime juice
    2 Tbsp. pure maple syrup
    1/10 Tsp. cayenne pepper
    Pure water — combine in 10 oz. hot or cold water
    Use 6 to 12 glasses daily
    You will not need anything else.

If you become constipated, taking an herb laxative in the morning and evening is helpful. Also use lemon skin or pulp with the cleansing drink. Use mint tea to neutralize odors from the mouth.

Cleansing Diet No. 2

Colon Cleanse the Easy Way by Vena Burnett and Jennifer Weiss

Cleansing Diet No. 3

Dr. Christopher's Three-Day Cleansing Program and Mucus-less Diet

Cleansing Diet No. 4

CLEANSING DIET FROM THE SENECA INDIANS — from *Good Health Through Diets* by Hanna Kroeger

FIRST DAY — eat fruit-all you want, such as apples, berries, watermelon, pears, cherries, but no bananas.

SECOND DAY—drink all the herb teas you want-such as Chamomile, Raspberry, Spearmint, Hyssop. If you sweeten it, use pure maple syrup.

THIRD DAY — eat all the vegetables you want-have them raw, steamed, or both.

FOURTH DAY — make a pan of vegetable broth using caulif-lower, cabbage, onion, green pepper, parsley or whatever you have on hand. Season with sea salt or herb seasoning. Drink only the rich mineral broth all day.

The reason this diet is beneficial is the first day the colon is cleansed. The second day you release toxins, salt and excessive calcium deposits in the muscle, tissue and organs. The third day the digestive tract is supplied with healthful, mineral rich bulk. The fourth day the blood, lymph and organs are mineralized.

GALL BLADDER CLEANSE FROM AUSTRIA

First Day — no food to be taken

8 a.m.	1 glass (8 oz.)	fresh apple juice
10 a.m.	2 glasses (16 oz.)	fresh apple juice
12 a.m.	"	"
2 p.m.	"	"
4 p.m.	"	"
6 p.m.	"	"

Second day — same as first day

At bedtime take 4 oz. of olive oil. Use lemon juice or hot apple juice to wash the oil down. Retire. It should start to work in the early morning. This helps dissolve the stagnant bile and liquifies through the malic acid of the apple juice. The oil moves the residue.

SECTION X

Fasting

Fasting is one of the oldest ways of healing and cleansing the body of diseases and build-up of mucus and toxins.

JUICE FASTING — Juice fasting helps restore the body to health as well as rejuvenates the system. It eliminates dead cells and toxic waste products that cause sickness and sluggish feelings.

Juice fasting is safer than a water fast because poisons in the body are released into the blood stream more slowly.

Some people fast anywhere from three to ten days.

Enemas are suggested during juice fasting by some nutritionists for it helps assist the body in its cleansing and detoxifying effort by washing out all the toxic wastes from the alimentary canal.

Fasting is very beneficial, but it must be remembered that during a prolonged fast, the body is cleansing itself without any opportunity to replenish or regenerate the cells and tissues. (Read—*Discover Your Fountain of Health* by Norman W. Walker, D.Sc., Ph.D, originator of fresh Vegetable Juice Therapy). The system is depleted of some of it's most vital essential elements.

Dr. Walker says that the immediate results of prolonged fasting is a feeling of well-being, but the damage on the system may not show up for one or two years or longer. Therefore the safest way to fast would be to go on fruit juices for three to four days at a time, or no longer than six days, and then break the fast by drinking vegetable juices to build the body and also by eating raw vegetable and fruits for two or three days.

This procedure can be repeated as long as it is felt necessary, but be sure and not fast more than six days.

A Green Drink is cleansing and can be used to prepare for a fast. It is nourishing and very high in chlorophyll. I use this drink when I feel a cold coming on or when I feel that my body is full of toxins.

In my green drink I use pineapple juice or fresh unfiltered apple juice, blended together with alfalfa sprouts, spearmint, parsley and comfrey.

My favorite juice diet is unfiltered apple juice for one, two, or three days at a time, and if I get hungry I eat apples in between drinking the juice. Before going to bed I use the Special Formula No. 1 and some type of laxative such as Cascara Sagrada.

A mild food diet should follow any fast. This way you don't overload the system with hard-to-digest foods.

Mild Food Diet

A mild food diet is used in chronic sickness and for periodic cleansing. The following foods are recommended:

Fruits, raw
Fruit juices, dilute half with pure water
Vegetables, raw, just steam lightly ones you cannot eat raw
Vegetable juices
Raw cold pressed oils, avoid rancid oils as they destroy vitamins and minerals
Raw nuts, keep in freezer to avoid going rancid
Honey, raw
Pure maple syrup
Seeds, sunflower, sesame and pumpkin
Sprouts (alfalfa, bean grain), use often for enzyme and vitamins, minerals, and chlorophyll
Bake all starch vegetables such as potatoes, squash, parsnips, yams and turnips

The following foods should be avoided during illness:

Grains, sugar, dairy products, butter, eggs, dried legumes, meats, peanuts, chips, soft drinks, including diet drinks

Foods to Eat

FRESH RAW FRUITS — Especially eaten in the season, where they are grown, Nature's cleanser and healer, full of vitamins and minerals.

FRESH RAW VEGETABLES — Eat as many raw as possible or steam lightly.

FRESH RAW FRUIT JUICES — Wonderful used in a fast, full of nutrients.

FRESH RAW VEGETABLE JUICES — Living food, full of enzymes, vitamins and minerals.

YOGURT, KEFIR, COTTAGE CHEESE PRODUCTS — Made with certified raw milk when possible.

KELP — Contains iodine, use instead of salt.

CHEESES — Made naturally without artificial coloring and synthetic processing.

SEEDS — Ground up or sprouted, important to have sprouts on hand as they are living foods.

NUTS — Raw and fresh, keep in freezer to keep from getting rancid.

WHOLE GRAINS — Freshly ground when ready to use or sprouted for live enzymes.

HONEY — Pure and natural, raw, full of vitamins and minerals, easily assimilated.

PURE MAPLE SYRUP — Contains vitamins and minerals.

COLD PRESSED OILS — Contains Vitamin E, use with lemon juice or pure apple cider vinegar, use on salads.

FERTILE EGGS — Contains protein and vitamins.

HERBS — Use garlic, capsicum, parsley, watercress, and paprika often.

DRIED FRUITS — Must be dried naturally in the sun with no chemicals added, should be soaked in water before eating to be more effective.

NATURAL SAUERKRAUT — Made at home fresh without chemicals with no salt added, very rich in calcium, and has great curative value.

HERBAL TEAS — Chamomile, licorice, spearmint and red raspberry

Natural Foods

ALMONDS — High in protein, Vitamin E., calcium.

APPLES — Protein, enzymes and minerals. Useful for whatever ails you.

APRICOTS — Minerals, especially iron. Detoxifies the liver and pancreas. High in vitamin A. Good for blood and skin, destroys worms.

AVOCADOS — High in protein and fat. Good for the diabetic and hypoglemiac.

BERRIES: —

BLACKBERRIES — good for the colon and diarrhea.

BLUEBERRIES — nourishes the pancreas.

STRAWBERRIES — Good for the skin, cleans the body and removes metallic poisons such as arsenic.

CAROB POWDER — Alkaline, contains minerals, a natural sweetner.

278

CHERRIES — Cleanses intestines, minerals. Eat in season for one cleansing food diet. Also drink cherry juice.

CITRUS FRUITS — Vitamin C, use lemons, limes and pure water on occasional fasts. Cleanser, eliminates toxins. Juice of three lemons or limes in quart of warm water to drink during a fast. Helps eliminate the flu.

COCONUTS — Supplies roughage.

DATES — High in protein, iron and mineral content, calcium and potassium.

FIGS — Contain iron, minerals, good for constipation.

FRUITS — All fruits, very nourishing, especially when eaten in the season. Cleans and builds the body.

GRAINS — concentrated foods, Buckwheat, Barley, Millet, Oats, Rye and Wheat. High in protein. Food for the vegetarian.

GRAPES — Blood builder, good for anemia, anti-tumor food.

HONEY — High in vitamins and minerals, use as substitite for white sugar. Use pure honey.

MUSTARD SEEDS — Good for digestion and gas.

NUT BUTTER — More nourishing than dairy butter, grind fresh when ready to use.

NUTS OF ALL KINDS — Raw, protein, unsaturated fats, minerals. Almonds, cashew, pecans, pistachio and walnuts.

OILS — Cold pressed are needed to assimilate the proteins from vegetables. Considered a kidney food.

PAPAYA — Good for digestion. Especially for protein foods.

SEEDS — Contains the germ and embroyo. Rich in oil, vitamin E, vitmain B-complex, minerals and proteins.

SPROUTED SEEDS — Very healthy, the freshest food you can eat. Rich in enzymes, B-vitamins and hormones. Alfalfa, wheat, mung beans, radish, fenugreek, sunflower and chick peas.

SUNFLOWER SEEDS — Protein, vitamins and minerals. Feeds the eyes, sinuses and glands.

VEGETABLES — High in enzymes, vitamins and minerals, carrot juice diluted is very good.

WATERCRESS — Natural immune properties. High in vitamin A and C.

YOGURT — Beneficial for intestinal health.

Fitness with Mini Trampoline

Running is not for everyone—running on concrete can cause problems to the bones, joints, muscles and ligaments of the feet and lower legs. Calluses and corns may develop due to pressure on feet especially with improperly fitted shoes. Sprains and tears to the Achilles tendon are common complaints of the jogger, especially without proper warmups.

Backaches are a major problem of many people and jogging on hard surfaces seems to agravate them. Doctors have reported that one of the major causes of back problems (about 75 million Americans suffer back problems) is doing improper exercises and that includes jogging on hard irregular surfaces. Knee injuries and shin splints are also a major complaint.

A wonderful way to get into shape without the demands and joint trauma of jogging is by using a mini-jogger. The mini-jogger is for everyone. For good cardiovascular fitness, you should jump for at least twelve minutes. Jumping to music is fun. This is an excellent exercise for senior citizens. You can do an easy jog, jog-dance to music, imagining jump rope, or a figure-toning jog.

When you exercise regularly the heart will become stronger and pump more blood with each beat. The total amount of blood in the body will increase since more oxygen has to be carried to the cells and more carbon dioxide is carried away from the cells. The number of small blood vessels will increase in order to improve the blood supply to every cell. The blood vessels will become more elastic.

The more one exercises the better the cells and the body are supplied with blood. You will be more alert, your brain will function better, you will tire less easily. Exercise will burn calories, tone muscles, relieve emotional tension and create a sense of well being.

SECTION XV

Herbs for Pregnancy

The best thing a mother can do for her child is to obtain proper nutrition, exercise, fresh air, lots of pure water, sunshine, adequate sleep and relaxation.

About 80% of the diet should be raw, natural food. The best foods are:

GRAINS: Buckwheat, brown rice, millet and wheat (if there is no allergy)

NUTS: Almonds, filberts, pecans and pinenuts (they should be eaten raw)

SEEDS: Sunflower, flax, sesame and pumpkin

VEGETABLES: Green leafy vegetables are full of vitamins and minerals. Try to eat most of your vegetables raw. Potatoes, squash, yams, green beans and artichokes can be steamed. Sprouts are full of live enzymes. Alfalfa sprouts are the most nutritious. Try sprouting beans a few days before cooking

FRUITS: All fresh fruit in the season

DURING PREGNANCY

The one herb that is renown for pregnancy is RED RASPBERRY. It can be used as a tea or in capsule. It is safe and effective, strengthens the uterus for easier delivery and there is less bleeding. It is high in iron, helps in after pain and birth defects. Women who take Red Raspberry usually have shorter labors.

The following formulas are very helpful and can be taken during pregnancy.

No. 1   Kelp, Dandelion, Alfalfa.
No. 2   Red Beet, Yellow Dock, Strawberry, Lobelia, Burdock, Nettle, Mullein.

ANEMIA: Iron is essential for the formation of hemoglobin which carries the oxygen from the lungs to every cell of the body. Pregnant women need extra iron. The above two formulas are very useful. Add Yellow Dock (it is almost 50 % iron). Drink a green drink. The following is my favorite:

Use either raw apple juice or pineapple juice, then add comfrey, alfalfa sprouts, spearmint or peppermint leaves, parsley and wheat grass: blend in the blender.

Add Vitamin C, about 500 Mgs. it helps iron absorb. Vitamin E strengthens the blood cells.

CONSTIPATION: Eat raw vegetables and fruits daily. Brewer's yeast and yogurt are useful. Use bran daily, always drink a large glass of water with bran, or it could cause further constipation. Psyllium or a lower bowel herbal formula is helpful.

FALSE LABOR: Drinking catnip as a tea in small amounts will help. Blue cohosh is known to help relax the uterus.

GAS: Fresh papaya or papaya tablets will help. Small amounts of ginger are also helpful.

HEARTBURN: Papaya tablets will help. Comfrey and pepsin combination will also help.

INSOMNIA: Extra calcium will help. Add more yogurt to the diet. The following herbal combinations will help:

No. 1 Comfrey, Alfalfa, Oat Straw, Irish Moss, Horsetail, Lobelia.
No. 2 Comfrey, Horsetail, Oat Straw, Lobelia.

Take Chamomile tea with Calcium formula before going to bed. These combinations will also help leg cramp.

MORNING SICKNESS: Red Raspberry tea, catnip tea, peppermint or spearmint will also help. Digestive enzymes. Green Drink has helped some people. Alfalfa and peppermint tea have helped some people. Ginger. Herbal Essential oils have also been helpful.

MISCARRIAGE: Red Raspberry tea helps prevent miscarriage. Dr. Christopher's Uterine tonic, to prevent miscarriage: Wild Yam, Squaw Vine, False Unicorn, Cramp bark. Lobelia and capsium will help relax the uterus. Bayberry and Catnip help prevent miscarriage.

TOXEMIA: Green Drink is helpful to clean the blood stream. Alfalfa, raspberry and comfrey tea is also cleansing and nourishing to the body. The following combinations are useful:

No. 1 Kelp, Dandelion, Alfalfa.
No. 2 Red Beet, Yellow Dock, Strawberry, Lobelia, Burdock, Nettle, Mullein.
Stay away from red meat, white sugar products and white flour products. Add more vitamins A and C to diet.

SIX WEEKS BEFORE DELIVERY: The following formula will help the delivery and labor easier:

No. 1 Black Cohosh, Squaw Vine, Lobelia, Pennyroyal, Red Raspberry.
No. 2 Black Cohosh, False Unicorn, Squaw Vine, Blessed Thistle, Lobelia, Pennyroyal, Red Raspberry.

CALCIUM FORMULAS:

No. 1 Alfalfa, Comfrey, Horsetail, Irish Moss, Lobelia.
No. 2 Comfrey, Horsetail, Lobelia, Oat Straw.

Calcium formulas will help build strong bones and teeth, it helps calm the nerves, and gives the mother sufficient calcium.

Nursing Mothers

NURSING: Blessed Thistle is known to increase mother's milk. Brewer's yeast taken daily will increase milk as well as give the mother necessary energy. Red Raspberry and Marshmallow tea is good. Alfalfa is excellent for rich milk and strength for the mother. Fennel Seed boiled in barley water helps increase mother's milk.

BREASTS: First signs of breast becoming infected, take 1000 mgs. of Vitamin C every hour. Take extra Vitamin A and E and garlic capsules. Green Drink is helpful for infections.

Cracked: Apply thin honey or almond oil. Helps prevent soreness and cracked nipples.

DRY UP MILK: Parsley and sage will dry up mother's milk.

Herbs for Children

FIRST YEAR OF LIFE: Fruit and vegetable juices or nut milks, always diluted. Raw apple juice and fresh carrot juice are very nourishing. Vitamin C must be given: Needed daily to build up resistance to germs. Babies need the amino acid (building blocks for body tissues) Taurine and mother's milk has a good supply but synthetic formulas don't. A deficiency of this amino acid in experiments has induced epileptic seizures. Taurine and B6 is a good combination for seizure problems.

COLIC: Catnip tea has been used for years for colic in babies. Fennel and peppermint tea are good. Tincture of Lobelia may be added to the tea.

CONSTIPATION: Small amount of mullein added to warm water, weak licorice tea is good for babies. The nursing mother should watch her diet.

CRADLE CAP: Vitamin E or Almond Oil rubbed into scalp.

DIGESTION: Difficulty in digesting cow's milk in children add powdered apple to milk or papaya. Fennel tea and Catnip tea.

DIAPER RASH: Ground comfrey, golden seal and make a paste with Aloe Vera juice. Vitamin E and A are good.

DIARRHEA: Carob flour in pure water every few hours. Barley water. Carob in boiled milk is good. Herb teas: Red Raspberry, Slippery Elm, Ginger, Strawberry, Sage, Yarrow and Oak Bark tea.

DRY SKIN: Olive oil, Vitamin A and E and Almond Oil. Aloe Vera is good.

EAR INFECTION: Garlic oil in ear. Garlic capsule in the rectum. Mullein oil, and Lobelia extract.

FEVER: Catnip tea, red raspberry or spearmint tea. Enemas help to bring fevers down.

HYPERACTIVITY: Keep children away from sweets, artificial coloring, flavoring and perservatives. B complex in water or juice. Calcium herbal formula. Vitamin D. Multiple vitamin and mineral tablet.

PINWORMS: Raisins soaked in senna tea for older children is an old time remedy. Chamomile and mint tea helps. Garlic in child's rectum will discard worms.

RESTLESSNESS: Chamomile tea, Lobelia extract rubbed on the back. Few drops of Lobelia extract on the tongue will help relax body.

TEETHING: Restless, crying babies who are teething need more calcium and vitamin D. Weak warm tea of catnip, chamomile, peppermint or fennel will help. Licorice root to chew on, it can dull the pain and irritation which teething causes.

SORE GUMS: Rub the gums with thick honey to which a pinch of salt has been added. Honey with oil of Chamomile, Lobelia extract rubbed on gums and Peppermint oil rubbed on gums will help.

URINATION PROBLEMS: Infants who cannot urinate: Crushed watermelon seeds made into a tea is beneficial. Small amounts given often.

Emergency Aids Plus Therapy Through Amino Acids

ALCOHOLISM — The amino acid Tyrosine in addition to tryptophan, niacin, vitamin B₆, hops, valerian and passion flower does as much for the alcoholic as do drugs and without the side effects.

Hops — good for delirium
Cayenne — reduces dilated blood vessels
Cabbage — helps sober
Golden seal — natural antibiotic
Chaparral — helps clean the residue of alcohol
Bee pollen — gives nourishment and strength to the body
Glutamine (amino acid) has been used in large doses to reduce the craving for alcohol

ALLERGIES — The best natural antihistamine is to cut orange peels in small strips and soak in apple cider vinegar for several hours, drain and cook down in honey until soft but not the consistency of candy. Keep in refrigerator. Use as needed. Relieves stuffiness and clogged passages.

Tyrosine (amino acid) — allergies are treated with tyrosine, especially cases of hayfever from grass pollen.

ARTHRITIS — the amino acid Histidine is good for tissue growth and repair and is useful for its anti-inflammatory effect and is used in rheumatoid arthritis.

Proline (amino acid) — is used in multiple amino acid and vitamin formula for arthritis

ASTHMA — Acute attack, it has been claimed that a few drops of Lobelia extract in the mouth will relax and put a stop to the spasms. Pour 1 cup cold water over 1-2 teaspoons shredded Elecampane root. Let stand 8-10 hours. Reheat. Take very hot, in small sips. Can sweeten with honey. Use 1 cup twice a day.

BLEEDING —

Cayenne pepper — a small amount applied in the nose has stopped bleeding immediately, taken internally with water helps internal bleeding, also helps a bleeding cut

Plantain — powdered or leaf applied directly on wound, dampen first

Marigold — the tincture in boiled water applied to wash the wounds, very useful in bleeding conditions

Shepherd's Purse — works as a styptic, use as a tea and apply as a poultice to the wound

BLISTERS — The amino acid, Methionine helps heal rashes and blisters in babies with high ammonia content in their urine. The amino acid Lysine has helped heal fever blisters when given 500 milligrams of lysine daily, with acidophilus and yogurt.

BOILS —

Figs — fresh figs applied hot, it is also used for mouth sores

Honey — an antibiotic, apply with a small amount of comfrey powder, apply and it will help bring boils to a head

Slippery Elm — use the powder added to water to make a paste, healing as a poultice, can be used for wounds, boils and skin problems

BRONCHITIS — Comfrey, Mullein, Lobelia is good. Bowels must be opened, an enema is helpful.

Lobelia tincture — for immediate needs if there is shortness of breath or gasping, if the throat needs to be cleared of mucus, a few drops of lobelia tincture will relax the throat and bronchi

Hot steam baths followed by a cold one with cold towels will help

Irish Moss — good for chronic bronchitis

Cysteine (amino acid) has the ability to build white cell activity and helps build resistance for respiratory diseases such as chronic bronchitis, emphysema, and tuberculosis

BRUISES — Comfrey powder, golden seal mixed with aloe vera juice is very good for bruises.

Mullein — the oil of Mullein flowers and olive oil is good for bruises

St. John Wort — the flowers are infused in olive oil and applied to bruises and wounds

Shepherd's Purse — the whole plant as a poultice for bruises

Witch Hazel — used as a compress, dipped in distilled Witch Hazel is good for bruises and swellings

BURNS — immediately immerse in cool water, apply vitamin E oil and take vitamin E orally, other remedies are:

Aloe Vera plant — cut off leaves, slit leaf and squeeze
  juice or lay exposed side of leaf on burn
Wheat germ oil and honey — make a paste of wheat germ
  oil and honey in blender, letting it run at low speed,
  then add comfrey leaves to make a thick paste, apply
  to burn, keep remainder in refrigerator
Marshmallow compress — can be used for mild burns
Potatoes — peeled raw potatoes will help on burns
Vitamin C applied topically and taken internally reduces
  pain eliminating the need for morphine

CHAPPED HANDS — Apply aloe vera gel to chapped hands and chapped lips

CHICKEN POX — Catnip tea enema

External teas — red raspberry, catnip, peppermint with
  vinegar to relieve itching
Golden seal tea — for severe itching
Lemonade with honey — fresh vegetable and fruit juices,
  if possible

COLDS AND FLU — Use mild teas made from catnip
or peppermint or red raspberry, use boneset, elderberry
and peppermint teas for cases of the flu, give natural
vitamin C liquid.

Chamomile tea — relaxing and soothing for colds and flu
Lemon and honey water — steeped and used for colds and
  coughs, refreshing and restorative
Honey — added to herb drinks will help destroy bacteria
  for the honey is a bactericide
Barley water — wash 2 ozs. of barley and boil in 1 pint of
  water for a few minutes, discard water then place
  barley in 4 pints pure water, add clean lemon peel,

boil down to 2 pints, strain and add 2 ounces of honey, can be used freely for children

CONSTIPATION — Prevention is the best method, the diet for children should include whole-grain cereals, leafy greens, raw fruits with skins are essential in keeping the bowels working normally. Emotional disturbances in the mother affect the baby if nursing.

Chamomile tea — weak chamomile tea is good for constipation
Cascara Sagrada — small amounts for children.
Elder flowers — good in cases of constipation
Licorice added to herbal teas has a slight laxative action
Nursing babies are rarely constipated if the mother is taking bulk in her diet
Weak molasses water will help
Acidophilus and yogurt are good for constipation
Licorice tea is good for constipation in babies

CONVULSIONS — weak chamomile tea in small doses several times a day helps. A warm chamomile tea enema is helpful.
Lobelia tincture can also be rubbed well into the neck, chest and between the shoulders.

COUGHS — If the cause of the cough is in the lung area, a cleansing diet is helpful.

Onion remedy — peel, and chop onions, cover with honey. Simmer. Strain and use as a cough syrup.
Honey and licorice root or honey and horehound herb, or honey and wild cherry bark are useful
Mullein — good for croup cough
Combination of marshmallow, mullein, comfrey, lobelia and chickweed in equal parts are good for coughs
Pitted dates crushed and made into a syrup has been used for coughs, sore throat and bronchitis

Infant suffocating from phlegm — lobelia extract on tongue

Tea of sage and thyme in equal parts with a pinch of cardamon and ginger and cloves and nutmeg is another remedy for coughs

Heavy cough — cherry bark tea and colts foot flower tea

Chew on licorice or candied ginger

Almond drink — grind almonds into powder and steep in 1 pint of cold water, will soften coughs and is a nutritious drink for a fever

Horehound remedy — use 2 tablespoons of the fresh leaves with two cups of boiling water, drink in small amounts

CROUP — Bring perspiration by giving the child warm catnip or chamomile tea.

Peppermint and honey is good

A few drops of lobelia tincture in catnip or peppermint tea is helpful

For nourishment, slippery elm gruel with oatmeal is good

DEPRESSION — the amino acid, Tyrosine, has been found to have a fantastic effect on depression for its management and control and compared to a drug used for depression with one great difference, no side effects.

Gotu Kola — helps in mental fatigue which is common in depression

Ginseng — helps stimulate the entire body energy to overcome depression

Kelp — contains all the minerals for glandular health

Herbal combinations — black cohosh, capsicum, valerian, mistletoe, ginger, St. John's wort, hops, wood betony

DIARRHEA — it must be remembered that diarrhea is natural in times of fear and stress, it is nature's way of

quickly removing the toxins in the body. An occasional diarrhea is not alarming.

Red Raspberry tea is soothing for diarrhea
Carob Powder in boiled milk. Usually about 1 teaspoon to
    1 cup milk
Barley water given to small babies is good for diarrhea
Licorice or Ginger is good to help colic pains from
    diarrhea
Carrot soup — is an excellent remedy for infant diarrhea,
    the cooked soup coats the inflammed small bowel,
    soothes it, and help promote healing
Slippery Elm Tea — nourishing as well as healing
Ginger — a weak ginger tea settles the stomach and helps
    in diarrhea

DIPHTHERIA —

Pineapple juice, lemon juice and honey or cider vinegar
    and honey is useful
A pinch of cayenne can be used for older children
Pineapple juice will cut the mucus

EARACHE —

Oil of garlic in the ear — hold in with cotton
Oil of lobelia in each ear — hold in with cotton

EYE INFLAMMATION —

Lotion of eyebright or chickweed
Eyebright tea strained

FEVER — high fevers, an enema is needed to reduce the temperature.

Barley water for high fever — (use linen cloth to tie barley
    and boil for ½ hour)
Licorice water
Elderflower and peppermint leaves

HEADACHES — capsuled Hops with water — Wood Betony, Chamomile tea, Tei-Fu Oil rubbed on temples Severe headaches — fasting with juice and green drinks. Herb laxatives, senna or cascara sagrada

HEMORRHOIDS — ginger tea, yarrow extract, white oak bark. Applied externally.

HERPES SIMPLEX I — (fever blisters or cold sores)

Infects the tissues around the lips and inside the mouth. The amino acid, Lysine inhibits the virus, together with vitamin C, zinc and vitamin A

Yogurt and buttermilk will eliminate the pain — halt the spread of the lesions and promote healing

HERPES SIMPLEX II — (Transmitted through sexual contact)

Black walnut — used internally as well as externally

Golden seal — mixed with aloe vera for external use, internally to speed healing of infection

INSECT BITES AND BEE STINGS —

Clay — a clay paste dampened and applied to the bite and sting will help relieve the pain

Plantain — wet plantain leaf with a little olive oil and place on bee or hornet sting, after the stinger is removed will help to heal, you need to replace the leaf as it dries

Honey — apply honey after removing the stinger

Comfrey — mixed with aloe vera juice will heal bites and take down the swelling

INSOMNIA — Plain, warm milk contains generous amounts of the amino acid Tryptophan which quiets the

nervous system and when taken with vitamin B$_6$ keeps the Tryptophan high in the blood stream. It is an essential ingredient for the regeneration of the body tissues. This is a natural alternative to tranquilizers.

Hot Chamomile Tea
Hops — help relax the body
Herbal calcium combination helps
Passion Flower — excellent for insomnia
Valerian — can be used occasionally, prolonged use can
    cause depression in some people

KIDNEY STONES — Apple juice and lemon juice fasts with olive oil. See *Own Your Own Body* by Stan Malstrom

MEASLES — Hot catnip tea or chamomile tea will break out the rash and check the fever, three tablespoons of the herb in a quart of water and boiled down to one pint.

MEMORY — The amino acid, Glutamine has been used with safety given to children who can't learn or retain memory.

Gotu Kola has been used with children to improve their learning ability and concentration

MUMPS — hot catnip tea relieves pain. Scullcap, ginger, cayenne, Fenugreek tea.

RINGWORM — a fungoid parasite is best stopped by sealing off the air.

Undiluted lemon juice, white of egg, nail varnish — apply
    every few hours
Garlic internally is helpful
Apply tincture of lobelia and olive oil

SCARLET FEVER — saffron is good. Raspberry
tea. Calcium herb formula. Ginger baths.

SUNBURN — to avoid sunburn mix one teaspoon vinegar to ½ cup thin sun flower oil and apply.

Gel from aloe vera plant is useful for sunburn
Equal parts of honey and wheat germ oil with powdered
comfrey added. Make paste ahead and it will keep
well in a covered jar

TOOTHACHE —

Hot poultices will reduce the pain of toothache
Chamomile and hop tea will help relax the body
Oil of clove — just a temporary relief, close oil can be
mixed with zinc oxide powder to form a paste, this
will protect the cavity from food

TONSILLITIS —

Catnip tea enema — pineapple juice
Vegetable juices are useful in removing waste
Red raspberry tea — comfrey tea

WEIGHT CONTROL — The amino acid,
Phenylalanine, is effective in weight control because of its
positive effect on the thyroid.
Kelp — helps regulate the thyroid
Count calorie intake
Exercise every day
Fasting Formula — Licorice, Beet Root, Hawthorne and
Fennel

WORMS —

Grated raw apples sprinkled with anise seed in a salad will
get rid of worms

Cold sage tea is also good for worms

Garlic — excellent body cleanser

Papaya Latex is used in Asia for children to expel worms (obtain at health food stores)

Yarrow — tonic to the bowels after expelling worms

Pomegranate — good for pin worms, round worms and tape worms

Pumpkin seeds — help eliminate worms

Note*Brewer's yeast contains all of the amino acids listed

Herbal First Aid Kit

ALOE VERA GEL — excellent for burns and skin rashes, also used for insect bites and stings, poison oak and ivy, acne and itchy skin.

ANTISPASMODIC EXTRACT — contains Valerian, Anise, Lobelia, Black Walnut, Brigham tea, Licorice and Ginger, used for the nerves and spastic conditions, excellent in emergency conditions such as hysteria, shock, poisonous bites and stings, used externally for pain and muscular spasms.

CAPSICUM — powder and extract, can be rubbed on toothaches, inflammation and swellings, in treating arthritis, rub capsicum extract over the inflamed joint and wrap with flannel for the night. Is useful to stop bleeding internally and externally by helping to normalize the circulation. Capsicum and Plantain applied externally will draw out foreign bodies embedded in the skin.

CASCARA SAGRADA — safe tonic, laxative, very important to keep the bowels open in illness and avoid constipation.

CHAMOMILE — used as a tea, is safe for children in

colds, indigestion and nervous disorders, relieves menstrual cramps, externally, apply to swellings, sore muscles and painful joints.

CHARCOAL — used for diarrhea and intestinal gas, can be used as a poultice. Can be used in some poisoning.

CHLOROPHYLL — I keep liquid chlorophyll on hand for all kinds of emergencies. It is a good cleanser for the blood. It is good to clean the bowels. Good for children and nursing mothers. It is rich in minerals.

COMFREY — can be used for bleeding by using a strong decoction. It can be used internally and externally for healing of fractures, wounds, sores and ulcers, old time remedy from the Middle Ages as follows: place burned area in ice water until pain is gone, mix the following in blender: ½ cup wheat germ oil, ½ cup honey, and add as much dried or fresh comfrey leaves as it will take to make a thick paste and add a pinch of lobelia.

EUCALYPTUS OIL — useful for bronchial spasms, chills, colds, sore throat, rheumatism, good antiseptic and expectorant.

FLOWERS AND PLANTS, EDIBLE AND NUTRITIOUS — Chicory, Clover, Dandelion, Elderberry, Squash, Borage, Nasturtium Lamb's Quarters, Plaintain, Purslane, Rose Petals Violets and Wild Watercress.

FENUGREEK — dissolves mucus, good for infections of nose, throat and lungs. Helps to lower fevers. Excellent with comfrey for children.

GARLIC — powder and oil, "Nature's Antibiotic", the oil is used for ear aches, garlic taken with Capsicum and Vitamin C at the beginning of a cold will often help.

GINGER — excellent for upset stomach, nausea, colds and flu.

LOBELIA EXTRACT — can be used internally and externally to relax all spasms, a few drops in the ear will relieve earaches, Lobelia used with catnip as an enema is effective for fevers and infections, used externally in baths, compressions, poultices, and liniments for muscle spasms.

PEPPERMINT OIL — aids nausea, an excellent stomach aid, assists in digestion, cleanses and gives tone to the entire body, sedative for nervous and restless persons of all ages, promotes relaxation and sleep.

RED RASPBERRY — excellent for pregnancy, relieving nausea, prevents hemorrhage, reduces pain and eases childbirth, reliable for children for stomach problems, fevers, colds and flu.

SARSAPARILLA — a hot decoction, made with an ounce of root in a pint of water, will promote profuse sweating and will act as a powerful agent to expel gas from the stomach and intestines.

Body Systems Guide

Herbs have been used with success for centuries. It is the oldest form of therapy practiced by humans as well as animals. Millions of people have testified to the benefits of herbal medicine. Approximately eighty percent of the world's population today depends on medicinal plants to heal and prevent disease.

The world's population as well as physicians are turning more and more to herbal medicine because they are considered safer than drugs. The side effects associated with the use of drugs are too numerous to mention. Drug companies are being sued constantly and settle out of court to prevent publicity.

Americans are becoming educated and more involved in their own health. We, as individuals, realize we have to take responsibility for our own health. Drugs will not heal the body, they just cause more problems and suppress the disease further in the system. Good health comes through learning more about diet, herbs, vitamins, minerals, and supplements that protect as well as help the body heal itself.

In the past, doctors said herbs are unscientific, primitive, unproven, ineffective, possibly dangerous and do not have a place in our society today. This can no longer be said. There is now evidence of the validity of herbal medicine. Science can now prove why herbs work to help the body heal itself. They are natural and do not cause side effects. When used with knowledge and guidance herbs strengthen, clean, nourish and stimulate body functions and even prevent disease. We now know why the herbs work to heal the body.

Science has discovered the ingredients in herbs and now know why they work to prevent and heal diseases of the body.

ALFALFA — has been beneficial for arthritis and is rich in minerals that help prevent illness. We now know it contains antibacterial, anti-cancer and anti-rheumatic properties. It will also help in high cholesterol.

BLACK WALNUT — has been used for years to expel parasites, worms and as a blood cleanser for skin problems. It contains anthelmintic properties which is responsible for killing worms and parasites.

BURDOCK — has been known as one of the greatest blood cleansers. We now contribute it to its antibiotic and antifungal principles.

ECHINACEA — has been used traditionally in the treatment of infections and is now known to contain antibiotic properties.

GENTIAN — has been used in Europe for years for healing the digestive system. It is now known to contain ingredients that stimulate the gallbladder and pancreas, which promotes healing.

GOLDEN SEAL — has been used in Europe and in ancient America for infections. The berberine found in Golden Seal will kill infections. It will destroy giardia and other pathogen infestations.

GOTU KOLA — has been used for years as a blood

purifier and tonic by the Europeans. It contains asiaticoside which aids in skin diseases. It works well as a brain stimulant.

HOPS – has been valued as a a relaxant for centuries. It contains sedative properties to relax the nerves and supply nutrients to the nervous system.

With all the scientific evidence of the ingredients found in herbs we now know why nature provided us with these valuable plants. When used in their natural state they will not cause side effects, when used with prudence. Herbs have built-in ingredients that prevent side effects where drugs are derived from plants or man made and can cause numerous side effects.

SECTION XXI

The Circulatory System

Heart disease is the number one killer of adults in the United States. Nearly one million people die each year of heart disease and related cardiovascular illness. Heart disease is striking people younger each year without warning and often fatal. It hits in many cases, without chest pains, shortness of breath or other symptoms common in heart disease. Cholesterol collects around the heart first then accumulates in the veins and arteries.This is why the heart can suffer damage first without symptoms. These are related to bad diet, alcohol, smoking and lack of exercise. Life style and diet change should be considered in order to protect the circulatory system. A typical American diet of meat and potatoes, sugar, and white flour products is paving the way for heart disease. A proper diet of whole grains (high fiber), fresh vegetables and fruits and herbs will clean and nourish the arteries.

Poor bowel function is another important cause of accumulation of fats and other toxins on the artery walls. It creates stagnation in the bowels which fosters anaerobic bacteria which produce toxic waste. If the bowels are not properly eliminated after each meal, these toxins circulate in the blood stream and are deposited on the organs and other parts of the body.

311

Nutrients to help the Circulatory System

There are nutrients that support the circulatory system by cleansing, nourishing and strengthening the heart, blood, the arteries, veins and capillaries.

ORAL CHELATION FORMULA

A nutritional formula that cleans the entire system and helps the blood flow more freely, improves circulation so that proper nutrition and oxidation can function in the body. The natural chelating elements work in a bonding reaction and surround the plaque, much like a magnet attracts metals. The chelation elements remove the built-up deposits on the arterial wall.

The natural chelation formula contains vitamins, minerals, glandular extracts, amino acids and herbs. It contains chelated minerals, a process where they are absorbed better by the body. It contain l-cysteine, HCL, choline, PABA, l-methionine, fish lipids, citrus bioflavonoids, rutin, adrenal substance, spleen extract, thymus substance, inositol. Hawthorn berries and ginkgo biloba are two herbs beneficial for circulation. It contain vitamins A, D, E, C, B1,B2, B6, B12, Niacin, pantothenic acid, folic acid, biotin magnesium, iron, iodine, copper and zinc. It also contain chromium, selenium, potassium, manganese and calcium.

BLOOD PURIFYING FORMULAS

Impurities in the blood affect the heart. The toxins are collected by both the blood and the lymph fluid that pass through the heart continually. It is important to to purify the blood. The following formulas will help purify the bloodstream.

#1. Red Clover—Chaparral—Spice.

#2. This Chinese formula strengthens the blood, liver and glands.

Ganoderma—Dang Gui—Peony—Lycium— Bupleurum—Curcuma—Cornus—Salvia—Ho Shu Wu—Atractylodes—Achranthes—Ligustrum— Alisma—Astragalus—Ligusticum—Rehmannia— Panax Ginseng—Cyperus.

#3. This formula enriches the blood and strengthens the kidneys.

Pau D'Arco—Red Clover—Yellow Dock— Burdock—Sarsaparilla—Dandelion, Chaparral— Cascara Sagrad—Buckthorn—Peach Bark— Barberry— Stillingia—Prickley Ash—Yarrow.

CIRCULATORY SYSTEM ENHANCERS

#1. This formula will provide nutrients to the eyes, ears, and nose areas to clean and nourish.

Golden Seal—Bayberry—Eyebright—Red Raspberry.

#2. This formula increases resistance to stress with it natural nutrients to enhance the circulatory, glandular, and nervous systems.

Siberian Ginseng—Bee Pollen—Yellow Dock— Licorice—Gotu-Kola—Kelp—Schizandra—Barley Grass—Rosehips—Capsicum.

STRENGTHENS THE HEART AND CIRCULATORY SYSTEM

#1. This formula feeds and strengthens the heart.

Hawthorn Berries—Capsicum—Garlic.

#2. This Chinese formula is known to nourish the heart, and strengthen the circulatory system.

Schizandra—Dang Gui(Dong Quai)—Cistanche—Biota—Succinum—Ophiopogon—Cuscuta—Lycium—Panax—Ginseng—Polygonum—Hoelen—Dioscorea—Astragalus—Lotus—Polygala—Acorus—Zizyphus—Rehmannia.

#3. This stimulates circulation and elimination which has a positive affect on the immune system.

Garlic—Capsicum—Parsley—Siberian Ginseng—Golden Seal.

#4. This formula contain Ginkgo and Hawthorn. The Ginkgo protects the cells of the body and especially those of the brain. It increases circulation, to delivery oxygen and glucose to the cells. It protects against free radical damage, and protects the nervous system.

The Hawthorn improves coronary circulation, nourishes the heart, and helps to stabalize blood pressure.

#5. Capsicum, Garlic and Parsley are also beneficial to nourish the heart. Parsley is a natural diuretic, and rich in minerals. Garlic helps to dissolve cholesterol plaque on the artery walls. It stimulates lymphatic system to eliminate toxins and is a natural antibiotic.

#6. This formula is rich in iron for healthy blood.

Red Beet Root—Yellow Dock—Red Raspberr—Chickweed—Burdock—Nettle—Mullein.

Omega-3 EPA—An essential nutrient for the body. It helps the body create a hormone-type substance called prostacyclin. This prevents blood cells from sticking together and decreases the danger of blood clots producing strokes and heart attacks.

CoQ-10 Formula—Contains the minerals copper, iron, magnesium and zinc. Amino acids leucine, histidine and glycine and the herbs capsicum and hawthorn. This formula increases oxygen to the brain and cells, prevents circulatory problems. Strengthens the heart and immune system.

Liquid Chlorophyll—Repairs tissues. Helps to neutralize pollution that we eat and breathe. It helps in the assimilation of calcium and other minerals. Purifies and strengthens the entire body.

Suma, Astragalus, Siberian Ginseng, Ginkgo and Gotu Kola—A power house of herbs to increase circulation, feed and strengthen the brain, eyes, ears, nose and throat. Improves memory, alertness, and an overall good feeling of well-being.

L-Carnitine—Energizes the body, effective in lowering cholesterol, cleans the veins and arteries and strengthens the muscles, especially the heart. It burns fat, and reduces built-up fat in the body.cleans the veins and strengthens the muscles, especially the heart. It burns fat, reduces built-up fat in the body.

Single herbs for the Circulatory System:

Aloe Vera—Bilberry —Bugleweed—Butchers Broom— Cayenne—Cloves—Garlic—Ginger—Ginkgo—Hawthorn— Horseradish—Prickly Ash—Suma—Virginia Snake Root.

SECTION XXII

The Digestive System

Digestive disorders are one of the most common health problems people are plagued with today. Both the old and the young are having more digestive problems. Improper digestion can cause poor assimilation, especially essential minerals. Lack of minerals and essential fatty acids can produce unhealthy cells. Wrong food combinations, eating when under stress, overeating and digestive upsets causes fermentations and intestinal gases which are connected with cancer and other diseases. Digestive upsets are mainly caused by stress, constipation, faulty diet, drugs, alcohol and tobacco. Eating wholesome, natural food nourishes the digestive system and strengthens the whole body.

DIGESTIVE FORMULA

This formula is more than a digestive aid, it works with the liver, gall bladder, and spleen to promote normal function of the digestive system. This will also benefit the lymphatic and urinary systems. It helps in the production of bile which digests fat and prevents constipation. This help with gas and bloating, fluid retention, digestion and in the assimilation of nutrients.

 #1. Rose Hips—Barberry—Dandelion—Fennel—
   Red Beet Root—Horseradish—Parsley—

317

#2.   Protein Digestive Aid HCL ——HCL decreases as people
      age. It is essential for the breakdown of proteins, starches
      and many foods. Hydroclyric acid destroys harmful
      bacteria. Worms and parasites are destroyed by HCL.

#3.   Digestive Enzymes — Necessary for digestion of proteins,
      fats and carbohydrates. Enzymes are essential for proper
      digestion. All food needs enzymes to be broken down
      into simple building blocks. Enzymes are destroyed by
      heating, emotional stress, drugs and toxins we eat and
      breathe.

DIGESTIVE SYSTEM FORMULAS

These formulas improve digestion and most ailments are
benefited when digestion is strengthened. These herbs help to
calm a nervous stomach, aid digestion, provide enzymes and
protein digestive aids.

#1.   This is a Chinese formula which enhances the
      digestive system and also benefits the urinary system
      in the elimination of toxins. It will help prevent
      nausea, gas, bloating, allergies, motion sickness and
      craving for sweets.

Agastache—Magnolia—Shenqu Tea—Crataegus—
Oryza—Hoelen—Panax Ginseng—Pinellia—Saussurea—
Gastrodia—Citrus—Atractylodes—Cardamon—Platycodon—
Ginger—Licorice—

#2.   Papaya—Ginger—Peppermint—Wild   Yam—
      Fennel—Dong Quai—Spearmint—Catnip—

#3.   Barberry—Ginger—Cramp Bark—Fennel—Pepper-
      mint—Wild Yam—Catnip.

#4.   Red Beet Root—Dandelion—Parsley—Horsetail—
      Liverwort—Black Cohosh—Birch—Blessed Thistle,

Angelica—Chamomile—Gentian—Golden Rod.

#5. Papaya and Mint.

#6. Golden Seal—Juniper—Uva Ursi—Cedar Berries—
Mullein—Yarrow—Garlic—Slippery Elm—
Capsicum—Dandelion—Marshmallow—Nettle—
White Oak Bark—Licorice.

#7. This formula benefits the stomach and the intestinal
system. It helps prevent indigestion, infections,
inflammations, ulcers and toxic accumulation.

Slippery Elm—Marshmallow—Dong Quai—Ginger—Wild
Yam—

#8. This Chinese formula is very beneficial to the
digestive and nervous systems. This will benefit in
many health problems. When the nerves are
strengthened it fortifies the immune system. This also
benefits the urinary and intestinal systems.

Bupleurum—Peony—Pinellia—Cinnamon—Dang Gui(Dong
Quai) Fushen—Zhishi—Scute—Atractylodes—Panax
Ginseng—Ginger—Licorice—

#9. This is another beneficial Chinese formula that works
with the digestive system. This strengthens digestion
to prevent indigestion, colitis, poor circulation and
many health problems that go along with an
unbalanced center of digestion.

Panax Ginseng—Astragalus—Atractylodes—Hoelen—
Dioscorea—Lotus—Galanga—Pinellia—Chaenomeles—
Magnolia—Saussurea—Dang Gui(Dong Quai)—Citrus Peel—
Dolichos—Licorice—Ginger—Zanthoxylum—Cardamon—

#10. This combination will strengthen and heal the
digestive and intestinal systems.

Ginger—Capsicum—Golden Seal—Licorice

Single Herbs for the Digestive System—Alfalfa, provides
    essential minerals and aids digestion. Aloe Vera-heals
    and protects the mucous membranes, will heal ulcers
    and even scars from adhesions.Buchu heals the
    digestive tract, absorbs excessive uric acid and acts as
    a tonic. Capsicum, heals and stops internal bleeding,
    acts as a disinfectant and aids in digestion. comfrey,
    Fennel, Gentian, Ginger, Papaya, Parsley, Peppermint,
    Slippery Elm.

The Glandular System

The glandular or endocrine system consists of the pituitary gland, thyroid gland, parathyroid gland, thymus gland, sex glands (ovaries, testes), pancreas, hypothalamus and adrenal glands.

Along with the nervous system, hormones, the secretions of the glands of the glandular system, are the major means of cor**olling the body's activities. The glandular system has a direct effect upon mood, mind, behavior, immune defense, memory, control of metabolic rate, and control of blood sugar to name a few.

All the glands depend upon one another and work together synergistically. The glandular system is necessary for survival, a healthy system is essential for health.

An imbalance in any gland of the glandular system will cause enormous problems for the entire body. There are many problems that can happen because of glandular imbalance. Vitamins, minerals and herbs nourish and restore glandular health.

GLANDULAR FORMULA—This was formulated to nourish and strengthen the entire glandular system. The nutrients of vitamins, minerals and herbs are combined with necessary essential ingredients to stimulate proper hormone production and metabolism.

Vitamin A nourishes the thymus gland,as well as all the glands, to increase its size and anti-body production. Zinc protects the immune system and supports the T-cells. Low zinc intake decreases thymus growth. Lecithin breaks down fatty deposits, especially effective on the liver. Vitamin C nourishes and cleans all the glands and with the lemon bioflavonoids, helps protect the immune system. The minerals, especially the trace minerals in the herbs, are vital for glandular health. Kelp is rich in iodine and contains all esential minerals. Alfalfa is rich in minerals and eliminates uric acid from the body. Parsley is a natural diuretic and eliminates toxins such as uric acid. Dandelion stimulates bile production and benefits the spleen and pancreas. Licorice root strengthens the adrenals, pancreas and spleen.

Vitamin A (beta-carotene)—Vitamin C—Vitamin E—Zinc—Pantothenic acid—Manganese—Potassium—Lecithin—Licorice—Lemon bioflavonoids-Asparagus powder—Alfalfa—Parsley—Kelp—Black Walnut—Thyme—Parthenium—Schizand...—Siberian Ginseng—Dong Quai—Dandelion—Uva Ursi—and Marshmallow—

HERBAL FORMULAS FOR THE GLANDULAR SYSTEM—

#1. This formula enhances the glandular system. It is especially beneficial for the pancreas in the production of pancretin and bile from the gallbladder. It also helps improve liver function, and is also beneficial for the urinary system.

Cedar Berries—Burdock—Chaparral—Golden Seal—Siberian Ginseng.

#2. This formula strengthens the digestive system. Lack of proper digestion can cause malfunction of the glands.

Barberry—Ginger—Cramp Bark—Fennel— Peppermint—Wild Yam—Catnip—

#3. This formula nourishes the pancreas, liver, adrenals as well as the digestive system.

Licorice—Safflower-Dandelion—Horseradish—

#4. This formula provide nutrition especially for the thyroid, but is beneficial for all the gland because of the complete mineral content. The minerals help eliminate toxic metal and poisons from the body.

Irish Moss—Kelp—Black Walnut—Parsley— Watercress—and Sarsaparilla—

#5. This formula helps bile production to digest fat and prevent constipation.It nourishes the liver, gall bladder, digestive system, spleen, immune system as well as the glandular system.

Rose Hips—Barberry—Dandelion—Fennel—Red Beet Root—Horseradish—Parsley—

#6. This formula is designed to feed the liver. The liver is vital to detoxify the system. A healthy liver is important to the glandular system.

Red Beet Root—Dandelion—Parsley—Horsetail— Liverwort—

Black Cohosh—Birch—Blessed Thistle—Angelica— Chamomile—Gentian—Golden Rod—

#7. This formula nourishes the glandular system, especially the pancreas and prostate.

Golden Seal—Juniper—Uva Ursi—Cedar Berries— Mullein—Yarrow—Garlic—Slippery Elm— Capsicum—Dandelion—Marshmallow—Nettle— White Oak Bark—Licorice—

#8. This formula is rich in minerals to give nutritional support to the glandular system, especially the hypothalamus and thyroid glands.These contain chelated minerals for easy absorption to benefit specific body systems.

Zinc—Manganese—Kelp—Irish Moss—Parsley—Hops—Capsicum—

#9. This formula helps balance the glandular system.It is rich in iodine, iron, calcium and magnesium.

Kelp—Dandelion—Alfalfa—

#10. This is a formula to benefit the glandular system especially the thyroid, the master gland. The hops are added to control the stress of the system. Stress depletes nutrients, and this will add extra nutrients to protect the glands.

Kelp—Irish Moss—Parsley—Hops—Capsicum—

#11. This formula is designed to nourish the glandular, nervous and circulatory systems. This is a natural way to provide the body with nutrients that help it adapt to stress.

Siberian Ginseng—Bee Pollen—Yellow Dock—Licorice—Gotu Kola—Kelp—Schizandra—Barley Grass—Rosehips—Capsicum-

#12. This formula is to support the glandular system when the body is undergoing fasting or cleansing programs. It will help nourish, strengthen and fortify the glands when under stress.

Chickweed—Cascara   Sagrada—Licorice—Safflower—Parthenium—Black Walnut—Gotu Kola—Hawthorn—Papaya—Fennel—Dandelion—

#13. This formula is excellent for athletes. It provides the body with nutrients not only for athletes but for anyone who is active in physical stress. It could also help parents who are acitve with children.

Siberian Ginseng—Ho Shou Wu—Black Walnut—Licorice—Gentian—Fennel—Slippery Elm—Bee Pollen—Bayberry—Myrrh—Peppermint—Safflower—Eucalyptus—Lemon Grass—Capsicum—

#14. This formula is to help the body maintain a balance in weight control. Along with a high fiber diet, using whole grains, fruits and vegetables and natural supplements, this formula will help in weight control.

Licorice—Red Beet Root—Hawthorn—Fennel—

#15. This formula is for an overstressed body, where the glands become weakened and puts stress on the entire body. This will give the body nutrients essential for the energy it needs to function properly.

Suma—Astragalus—Siberian Ginseng—Ginkgo—Gotu Kola—

#16 This formula is designed to support the nutritional needs of the pancreas.

Chromium—Zinc—Golden Seal—Juniper—Uva Ursi—Huckleberry-Mullein—Yarrow—Garlic—Slippery Elm—Capsicum—Dandelion—Marsh-mallow—Nettle—White Oak—Licorice—

#17 This is a Chinese formula that is very beneficial to strengthen the glandular system. When the glands are out of balance it can cause a number of health problems.

Dendrobium—Eucommia—Rehmannia—Ophiopogon—Trichosanthes—Pueraria—Anemarrhena—Achyranthes—Hoelen—Asparagus—Moutan—Alisma—Phellondendron—Cornus—Licorice—Schizandra—

FEMALE GLANDS

Female Glandular Formula, contains vitamins, minerals and herbs to provide nutritional support and prevent deficiencies that cause emotional and physical symptoms and problems. This nutritional support will help prevent physical and mental stress which causes fatigue, depression, irritability, and chemical imbalance which can lead to a dependency on anti-depressent drugs.

It contains Vitamins A, C, B1, B2, Niacinamide, Vitamin D, E, B6, Folic acid, B12, Biotin, Pantothenic Acid,and minerals, Calcium, Iron, Iodine, magnesium, Zinc, Copper,Manganese, Chromium, Selenium and Potassium. It also contains Choline, Inositol, Bioflavonoids, and PABA. It also contains the following Chinese herbs: Dong Quai, Peony, Bupleurum, Hoelen, Atractylodes, Codonopsis, Alisma, Licorice, Magnolia, Ginger, Peppermint, Moutan, Gardenia and Cyperus.

FEMALE FORMULAS

#1. This is designed to help maintain the female glands as well as other glands. This will nourish and strengthen the reproductive glands and prevent menstrual pain, pre-menstrual tension, insomnia, menopausal symptoms, sexual disinterest and other problems that are caused by chemical imbalance.

Black Cohosh—Licorice—Siberian Ginseng— Sarsaparilla—Squaw Vine—Blessed Thistle—False Unicorn—

#2. This formula is designed to help prepare a woman for giving birth by strengtening the glands and reprodutive systems. This supplies nutrients to build a weakened body, to prevent menstrual disorders, morning sickenss, miscarriage, as well as menopausal symptoms.

Black Cohosh—Squaw Vine—Dong Quai—Butcher's Broom—Red Raspberry—

#3. This is formulated especially for the female reproductive organs and also benefits the glandular system. This is rich in herbs that contain vitamins and minerals that feed and strengthen the female glands.

Red Raspberry—Dong Quai—Ginger—Licorice— Black Cohosh—Queen of the Meadow—Blessed Thistle— Marshmallow—

#4. This is designed to strengthen the female reproductive system and the urinary system. This helps to prevent cramps, bloating, morning sickness, and menstrual disorders.

Golden Seal—Red Raspberry—Black Cohosh— Queen of the Meadow—Althea—Blessed Thistle— Dong Quai—Capsicum—Ginger—

#5. This is a nutritional herbal supplement to help balance hormones, prevent bad estrogen from accumulating, bloating, post partum problems, weakness in the veins, hemorrhaging, anemia and strengthen the urinary system.

Golden Seal—Capsicum—Ginger—Uva Ursi— Cramp Bark—Squawvine—Blessed Thistle—Red Raspberry—False Unicorn—

#6. A liquid formula for easy digestion and assimilation. It enhances nutritional support for the digestive and glandular systems.

Peppermint—Rose Hips—Hibiscus—Red Raspberry—

Single Herbs for the Female Glands: Black Cohosh, Blessed Thistle, Blue Cohosh, Dong Quai, Red Raspberry, Suma.

MALE FORMULAS

#1. A special formula for the prostate gland as well as for the glandular system. This will help balance hormones in the body. It helps to supply nutrients for inflammation and pain in the prostate gland.

Black Cohosh—Licorice—Kelp—Gotu Kola—Capsicum—Golden Seal—Ginger—Dong Quai—

#2. A special formula for the male reproductive system as well as benefical for the urninary system. Nutrients to help prevent kidney stones, inflammation, infections, impotence, edema, joint pain, prostatitis.

Capsicum—Golden Seal—Ginger—Parsley—Siberian Ginseng—Uva Ursi—Marshmallow—Eupatorium—

#3. This is especially formulated for the male reproductive system. It provides nutrients to nourish and strengthen the prostate. It helps prevent swelling, inflammation and prevent pain. This is important for older men, who need nutrients for proper function of the male glands.

Siberian Ginseng—Parthenium—Saw Palmetto—Gotu Kola—Damiana—Sarsparilla—Horsetail—Garlic—Capsicum—Chickweed—

#4. This formula is designed to help strengthen the glandular system, especially for the pancreas and prostate. It helps in infections, water retention and supplies circulation to prevent toxins from accumulating in the glands.

Single Herbs for the Male Glands: Black Walnut—Damiana—Ho Shou Wu—Sarsparilla—Saw Palmetto—Siberian Ginseng—American Ginseng—Suma—

SECTION XXIV

The Immune System

The Immune System is a network of body compounds that keep us safe from bacteria, viruses, yeast or fungi infections and other toxins which invade our tissues. The Immune System accumulates damage, and gradually becomes defective over many years and is implicated in the auto-immune diseases that are prevalent now. Diet and life-style have a profound effect on the immune system. Evidence has been produced that shows how stress, and how we cope with stress, are the main causes of illness.

Stress effects the body by depleting the adrenal glands. This causes a supressed immune system. This happens because the immune system requires enormous amounts of nutrients. The body also requires large amounts of nutrients and the average American diet does not supply the body's needs. Our food is processed, with added chemicals, food colorings, preservatives and taste enhancers. The natural food is processed and depleted of the vital vitamins such as B-vitamins and minerals that are essential for a healthy immune system.

Viruses are composed of living and non-living material. They can be frozen for years and if the immune system is weak, come to life. The virus inserts its genetic material through the cell wall. It then dissolves the wall and fuses with the contents of the cell, this multiplies and begins to do its damage.

IMMUNE FORMULA

This formula contains nutrients to protect and strengthen the immune system. It contains the necessary ingredients for a healthy well-functioning immune system to fight toxins, germs and viruses that constantly invade our bodies.

Vitamin A from fish oils and beta carotene. Vitamin C—Vitamin E—Zinc and Selenium. Barley grass Juice Powder—Wheat Grass Juice Powder—Asparagus Powder—Astragalus—Broccoli Powder—Cabbage Powder—Ganoderma—Parthenium—Schizandra—Siberian Ginseng—Myrrh Gum—Pau D' Arco.

Special Immune Formulas:

#1. This formula was designed to nourish and strengthen the immune system. It also protects the body against stress and gives the body a feeling of well-being. This will aid in healing as well as protect against viruses that cause auto-immune diseases.

Rose Hips—Beta Carotene—Broccoli Powder—Cabbage Powder—Siberian Ginseng—Parsley—Red Clover—Wheat Grass Powder—Horseradish.

#2. This formula is beneficial for the immune and circulatory systems. This helps protect against germs and viruses that cause illness.

Rose Hips—Chamomile—Slippery Elm—Yarrow—Capsicum—Golden Seal—Myrrh Gum—Peppermint—Sage—Lemon Grass—

#3. This not only strengthens the immune system but aids in digestion and the lumph system. It helps in fever, vomiting, motion sickness, chills, abdominal pain, and water retention.

Ginger—Capsicum—Golden Seal—Licorice—

#4. Germanium Formula. Germanium is an antioxidant which neutralizes free radicals to prevent them from damaging tissues in the body. Echinacea helps neutralizes toxins and rid them from the body.

Germanium—Echinacea—

#5 This formula aids the body from stress that weakens the immune system. It also is beneficial for the lymphatic and respiratory systems.

Parthenium—Yarrow—Myrrh Gum—Capsicum—

#6. This formula is an immune system enhancer. It helps purify the lymphatic and strengthen the digestive systems. It helps in infections, colds, flu and with swollen glands.

Parthenium—Golden Seal—Yarrow—Capsicum—

#7. This formula strengthens the eliminative system which can cause a weakened immune system. A weak immune system will open the door to all kinds of illness.

Golden Seal—Black Walnut—Althea (Marsh-mallow)—Parthenium—Plantain—Bugleweed—

#8. Red Clover Formula. This formula helps purify the and eliminate toxins, germs and viruses from the body. It is also useful in liquid form for easy assimilation for those who have faulty digestion.

Red Clover—Chaparral—Spice—

#9. This formula is designed to strengthen the immune system. This contains chelated minerals which are necessary to enzymes for the immune system such as superoxide dismutase(SOD).

Vitamin A (beta-Carotene)—Copper—Manganese—Zinc—

#10. This formula is designed to fortify and strengthen the body to protect against yeast infestations and other microorganisms that invade when the immune system is weak.This provides nutrients to strengthen and protect the immune system.

Caprylic Acid—Vitamin A—E—C—Pantothenic Acid—Biotin—Zinc—Selenium. It also contains the following herbs. Pau D' Arco—Garlic—Golden Seal—Yucca—Lemon Grass—Rose Hips—Hesperidin Complex—Citrus Bioflavonoids—

#11. This formula is designed to protect and build-up the immune system. It contains nutrients that a vital for the protection of the immune system. The minerals have been chelated to specific amino acids glutamine and glycine. This provides for better assimilation.

Vitamin A (Beta-Carotene)—Copper—Manganese—Zinc—Barley Green Juice Powder—

#12. A combination of Golden Seal and Parthenium in an extractform is designed to heal and strengthen the immune systemand protect against diseases. Golden Seal is the greatest healer in the herbal kingdom. It will heal and repair the entire digestive tract. Parthenium will help the lymphatic system to keep the body clean.

#13. This Chinese formula is carefully designed to strengthen the immune system. It protects against viral infections, and protects against germs.

Dandelion—Purslane—Indigo—Thlaspi—Bupleurum—Scute—Pinella—Ginseng—Cinnamon—Licorice—

#14. This Chinese formula is designed to increase circulation, which helps fight and prevent infections. It will strengthen the immune system by stimulating circulation, which is the key to a healthy body.

Astragalus—Panax Ginseng—Dang Qui (Dong Quai)—Rehmannia—Epimedim—Ganoderm—Eucommia—Lycium—Peony—Polygala—Ligustrum—Schizandra—Atractylodes—Hoelen—Achyranthes—Ophiopogon—Citrus Peel—Licorice—

#15. This formula is in an extract for quicker assimilation to quicker action. It strengthens the immune and nervous systems. This is useful to help fight infections, especially for all kinds of ear problems, such as ear infections, accumulation of wax in the ears, itching ears, and has been used for some types of hearing loss. It can also be used for throat infections.

Black Cohosh—Chickweed—Golden Seal—Desert Tea-Licorice—Valerian—Scullcap—

SINGLE HERBS FOR THE IMMUNE SYSTEM

Barley Juice Powder—Blue Vervain—Burdock— Chaparral—Echinacea—Ginkgo—Golden Seal—Parthenium—Pau D'Arco—Rose Hips—Suma—

SECTION XXV

The Intestinal System

The colon is the body's sewer system, and if not treated properly can accumulate toxic poisons, which are absorbed into the blood stream. This will then cause many diseases. Lack of fiber in the diet is the main cause of intestinal diseases. Years of poor diet cause bowel problems.

The small intestine is where most nutrition is absorbed. Stress can affect nutrients absorption and cause irritation of the small intestine.

The large intestine absorbs minerals and water. When the membrane of the large colon is unhealthy, it cannot assimilate and absorb the minerals and creates deficiency diseases. The health of the entire body is maintained when the intestinal system is working properly.

BOWEL FORMULA—This benefits the entire gastrointestinal tract. It supplies nutrients for a healthy colon. It strengthens and heals the stomach, nourishes and cleans the intestines, stimulates bile function and liver health. It dissolves and eliminates mucus from the intestinal tract. It contains nutrients for proper digestion and assimilation.

It contains betaine HCl, pepsin, pancreatin and bile salts for upper gastrointestinal system. It contains Psyllium Hulls, Kelp and Chlorophyll to clean and

335

nourish the lower bowels. It also contains Vitamin C, E and Beta-carotene, selenium and zinc. It contains Algin, Cascara Sagrada, Bentonite Clay, Apple Pectin, Marshmallow Root, Parthenium Root, Charcoal, Ginger, and Sodium Copper Chlorophyllin.

GYMNEMA FORMULA-Excellent for the digestive and glandular systems. Research on gymnema shows good results on nourishing the pancreas and helping with problems such as diabetes, obesity and glandular problems.

Brindall Berries—Gymnema Leaves—Marshmallow—Psyllium Hulls—

PUMPKIN SEED FORMULA—Good for parasites, cleans the colon, skin problems, removes toxins from the system, constipation, prostate, tumors, worms.

Pumpkin Seeds—Culvers Root—Cascara Sagrada—Violet—Chamomile—Mullein—Marshmallow—Slippery Elm—

LOWER BOWEL FORMULAS—The herbs in this formula tone, rebuild and strengthen the bowels. They will gradually clean and restore bowel function. Constipation causes poisons to accumulate in the blood and prevents food from being assimilated.

#1. This formula is designed to help the entire intestinal tract. This will enhance normal liver function. It strengthens the gall bladder, urinary and lymphatic systems.

Rose Hips—Barberry—Dandelion—Fennel—Red Beet Root—Horseradish—Parsley—

#2. This formula will help heal and restore normal lower bowel function. It wil also help purify the blood.

Cascara Sagrada— Buckthorn— Licorice—

Capsicum, Ginger—Barberry— Turkey Rhubarb –
Couch Grass—Red Clover—

#3. This formula is rich in fiber and minerals for the lower bowels. It helps restore normal function to weakened bowels.

Dong Quai— Cascara Sagrada—Turkey Rhubarb—
Golden Seal—Capsicum—Ginger—Barberry—
Fennel—Red Raspberry—

4. This formula contains nature's natural fibers. It will absorb toxins and rid them from the body. It will help lower cholesterol. It is a natural way to restore normal bowel function.

Psyllium—Oat—Apple Fibers.

5. This formula is an excellent way to clean the bowels. The ginger helps prevent any cramps due to the Senna. The Catnip helps relax the bowels, and the formula is rich in minerals, which are absorbed in the lower bowels.

Senna Leaves— Fennel— Ginger—Catnip—

#6. This formula works on the lower bowels to promote the friendly bacteria, essential for a healthy colon. This is soothing and healing to the entire intestinal system.

Slippery Elm—Marshmallow—Plantain—
Chamomile—Rosehips—Bugleweed—

#7. This Chinese formula helps detoxify and clean the intestinal system.

Ionicera—Scute—Forsythia—Platycodon—
Ligusticum—Schizonepeta—Peony—Chrys-
anthemum—Gardenia—Phellodendron—Siler—
Bupleurum—Dang Qui (Dong Quai)—Arctium—
Vitex—Licorice—Carthamus—Coptis—

GENERAL CLEANSING FORMULA—This formula benefits
the colon, blood and cells of the body. It is an
excellent formula to use on a weight loss program. It
is an excellent blood cleanser to use for any disease.

1. Gentian—Irish Moss— Cascara Sagrada— Golden
Seal—Slippery Elm—Fenugreek—Safflower—
Myrrh—Yellow Dock-Parthenium—Black Walnut—
Barberry—Dandelion—Uva Ursi-Chickweed—
Catnip—Cyani—

SUPPLEMENTS FOR THE INTESTINAL SYSTEM—
Acidophilus—Aloe Vera Juice—Hydrated
Bentonite—Liquid Chlorophyll—Magnesium—

SINGLE HERBS—Black walnut—Buckthorn—Cascara
Sagrada—Chaparral—Dandelion—Fennel—
Fenugreek-Flax—Ginger—Golden Seal—Licorice—
Marshamllow—Oregon Grape—Peppermint—
Psyllium—Safflowers—Sarsparilla—Senna Vervain—
Slippery elm—

SECTION XXVI

The Nervous System

The nervous system is a very delicate and important part of the body and needs to be treated and fed properly. The nervous system and the immune system are closely connected. When one system fails the other is affected. The brain has the job of transmitting information back and forth from the immune system. It is vital to nourish and strengthen the nervous system in order to protect the immune system.

STRESS FORMULA—Stressful situations leach out nutrients from the body.Nutritionst regard inadequate nutrients as the most stressful on the immune system as well as the nervous system. This formula is designed to fortify the body against depleted essential nutrients and protect the body under stress.

It contain Vitamin C—B$_1$—B$_2$—B$_6$—B$_{12}$—Folic Acid—Biotin—Niacinamide—Pantothenic Acid—Schizandra—Choline Bitartrate—PABA—Wheat Germ—Bee Pollen—Valerian Root—Scullcap—Inositol—Hops—Citrus Bioflavonoids—

HERBAL FORMULAS FOR THE NERVES

#l.   This formula is designed to relax the nerves and nourish and strengthen the nervous system. It is especially good for spastic colon and muscle spasms. It helps prevent migraine headaches. It is rich in calcium and B-complex vitamins which provides nutritional support for the nervous system.

Chamomile—Passion Flowers—Hops—Fennel—Marshmallow-Feverfew

#2. This formula is designed to strengthen weakened nerves and help in nervous tension, cramps, headaches, hysteria, pain and insomnia. This will build the nerves to help in coughs, cramps, vertigo, and with colds, flu and fevers.

White Willow—Valerian—Lettuce Leaves—amd Capsicum—

#3. A formula to strengthen the nervous system as well as cleansing power to clean the muscles and tissues. The Devil's Claw works similar to Chaparral and enhances this formula.

White Willow—Black Cohosh—Capsicum—Valerian—Ginger—Hops—Wood Betony—Devel's Claw—

#4. This is formulated for an overstressed nervous system. To help in insomnia, hypertension, menstrual disorders, nervous indigestion, headache, epilepsy, arthritis and rheumatism.

Valerian—Scullcap—Hops—

#5. This formula not only strengthens the nervous system but benefits peripheral blood circulation. It helps relieve anxiety and tense muscles. It will gradually build a strong nervous system which protects the immune system. Valerian is rich in calcium and the passion flower is beneficial for the eyes.

Black Cohosh—Valerian—Capsicum—Passion Flower—Scullcap—   Hops-Wood Betony—

#6. This Chinese formula is beneficial on the nervous system. It helps to prevent depression, insomnia, fatigue, anxiety, and menopause symptoms. It also strengthens the urinary, respiratory and female reproductive systems.

Perilla—Saussurea—Gambir—Bamboo Sap—Bupleurum—Pinellia—Aurantium—Zhishi—Ophiopogon—Cyperus—Platycodon—Liqusticum—Dand Gui—Panax—Ginseng—Hoelen-Coptis—Ginger—Licorice—

#7. An extract formula which is used to calm, nourish, and strengthen the nervous system. It is useful for those who need to build up their digestive system. It is easily assimilated and contains minerals to build up the digestive and nervous system. It can be used under the tongue with quick results.

Valerian—Anise—Black Walnut—Desert Tea—Ginger—Licorice—

#8. This Chinese formula contains nutrients vital for a strong nervous system. It also benefits the digestive and urinary systems.

Dragon Bone—Oyster Shell—Albizzia—Polygonum—Fushen—Polygala—Acorus—Panax Ginseng—Saussurea—Zizphus—Curcuma—Haliotis Shell—Coptis—Cinnamon—Licorice—Ginger—

#9. This combination supplies nutrients that strengthen the nervous system. It also benefits the respiratory and muscle systems.

Blessed Thistle—Pleurisy—Scullcap—Yerba Santa—

Shattered nerves are in need of the B-complex vitamins and an herbal calcium formula. Vitamin C with bioflavonoids are essential for the healing of the nerve sheath which surrounds the raw nerves.

SINGLE HERBS FOR THE NERVES—

Bilberry—Black Current Oil—Catnip—Chaparral—Feverfew—
Hops— Lady's Slipper—Passion Flower—Scullcap—
Valerian—Wood Betony—

SECTION XXVII

The Respiratory System

Respiratory infections are the most frequent single cause of illness. one-third to one-half of industrial absenteeism from sickness is caused by acute respiratory illness. The lungs have the responsibility of supplying oxygen necessary for body energy.

Toxins present in the atmosphere, such as nitrogen and ozone dioxide, are increasing as a major cause of respiratory problems. Pollutants can attack the body repeatedly over a long period before symptoms appear. The respiratory system consists of the lungs, nose, throat and trachea.

Herbs, vitamins, minerals and proper diet will help keep the respiratory system strong and healthy. A colon cleanse is essential for a healthy respiratory system.

RESPIRATORY FORMULA

This formula was developed for severe lung congestion, allergies, lungs filling with fluid, mucus, pneumonia, coughs and toxic build-up in the lungs. It also helps in digestion. The herbs in this formula will help protect the lungs from all the pollutants in the air. It helps loosen hard mucus from the sinuses, throat, and lungs. It will help in asthma, bronchitis, coughs, hayfever, nasal drainage, earache, sinus swelling and swollen glands.

Boneset—Fenugreek—Horseradish—Mullein—Fennel—

SPECIAL RESPIRATORY FORMULAS

#1. This Chinese formula is beneficial for the respiratory system. It also helps with the circulatory and lymphatic systems. It increases circulation and eliminates toxins from the system.

Citrus Peel—Pinellia—Ma Huang—Fritillaria—Bamboo Sap—Bupleurum—Hoelen—Platycodon—Xingren—Morus—Magnolia—Tussilago—Ophiopogon—Schizandra—Ginger—Licorice—

#2. These two combinations are very beneficial for the respiratory system. Fenugreek and Thyme are especially beneficial for the sinuses and head area. They both help prevent and eliminate mucus from the respiratory system. It helps keep the lungs and the nasal passages clean to prevent germs and viruses from multiplying.

Fenugreek—Thyme—

Marshmallow—Fenugreek—Slippery Elm—

#3. This formula is designed for the nervous and muscle system as well as the respiratory. This supplies nutrients to heal and strengthen the respiratory system.

Blessed Thistle—Pleurisy—Scullcap—Yerba Santa—

#4. This formula is excellent for the lungs. It supplies nutrition for the respiratory system. This helps in asthma, allergies, coughs, sinus headache and sinus irritation that causes drainage in the throat.

Marshmallow—Chinese Ephedra—Mullein—Passion Flower—Catnip—Senega--Slippery Elm—

#5. This formula is designed for the entire respiratory system and is especially effective for the sinuses.

It helps clean and strengthen the mucous membranes of the nose, throat and lungs to prevent allergies and other respiratory problems.It helps with hay fever, sinus irritations, itching eyes, irritating coughs, asthma, bronchitis and respiratory infections.

Chinese Ephedra—Senega—Golden Seal—Capsicum—Parsley—Chaparral—Burdock—

SINGLE HERBS FOR THE RESPIRATORY SYSTEM

Angelica—Boneset— Comfrey— Ephedra—Fenugreek—Flaxseed— Golden Seal—Licorice—Lobelia—Marshmallow—Mullein—Yerba Santa—

The Structural System

The structural system consists of bones, muscles and connective tissue. Poor nutrition and the inability to assimilate minerals, contribute to bone loss. High protein and sugar diets, smoking, alcohol, caffeine drinks, and lack of exercise all contribute to bone loss as well as pave the way for other diseases.

Bone loss in women after menopause is a special concern. This is when decreased secretion of the hormone estrogen is greatest. This isn't necessary if a balanced diet is followed with ample supply of minerals. The ability to assimilate minerals is a concern seen in the young as well as the elderly.

STRUCTURAL FORMULA

This formula is disigned to provide nutrition for the bones, flesh and cartliage of the structural system. There are many nutrients that contribute to a healthy structural system, and the following have been beneficial.

Vitamin A (beta-carotene)—Vitamin C—Calcium(chelated for easier assimilation)—Iron—Vitamin D—B_6—B_{12}—

Phosphorus— Magnesium—Manganese—Potassium—
Horsetail—Betaine HCI (necessary for the assimilation of
calcium and other minerals)—Papaya— Parsley—Pineaple—
Valerian—Licorice—Ma Huang—

Special Structural Formula

This formula will strengthen and nourish the
structural system. Copper, potassium and zinc chelated to
the amino acids argine, leucine and glycine. It contains
Bee Pollen—Siberian Ginseng—Gotu Kola—Capsicum—
Licorice—Glutamine—Choline Bitartrate.It also contains B$_6$—
B$_{12}$—Vitamin C—Calcium—Copper—Folic Acid-Iodine—
Niacinamide—Pantothenic acid—Potassium—Phosphorus—
Zinc—

Special Structural Formulas

#1. This formula strengthens the structural, nervous and
immune systems. This helps prevent arthritis, gout and
rheumatism as well as other related problems.

Bromelain—Hydrangea—Yucca—Horsetail—
Chaparral—Alfalfa—Black Cohosh—Catnip—
Yarrow—Capsicum—Valerian—White Willow—
Burdock—Slippery Elm—Sarsaparilla—

#2. This is especially beneficial for increasing bone mass
as well as strengthening the nervous system. It is rich
in calcium as well as minerals to help in the
assimilation of calcium.

Alfalfa—Marshmallow—Plantain—Horsetail—
Oatstraw—Wheat Grass—Hops—

#3. This is formulated to nourish the hair, skin and nails. It
is a benefit to the structural system. It is rich in
silicon, which has shown to be beneficial to calcium

assimilation to strengthen the bones and the entire body.

Dulse—Horsetail—Sage—Rosemary—

#4. This is a formula to use internally and externally. It will heal and rebuild tissues. It will help in cases of adhesion, which cause a lot of pain and misery.

Slippery Elm—Marshmallow—Golden Seal—Fenugreek—

#5. This Chinese formula is designed to strengthen the bones. It also helps enhance the urinary system. It helps in backaches, fatigue, arthritis, osteoporosis and tones up the structrual system.

Eucommia—Cistanche—Rehmannia—Morinda—Drynaria—Achyranthes—Hoelen—Dipsacus—Lycium—Dioscorea—Ligustrum—Cornus—Dang Gui(Dong Quai)—Panax Ginseng—Astragalus—Epimedium—Liguidambar—Atractylodes—

SINGLE HERBS FOR THE STRUCTURAL SYSTEM

Aloe Vera—Bayberry—Comfrey—Horsetail—Oatstraw—Red Raspberry—White Oak Bark—Yucca—

SECTION XXIX

The Urinary System

The Urinary System consists of the kidneys, bladder, ureters and urethra. Keeping this system in good working condition will help prevent the body from poisoning itself. The proper function of this system is vital to our inner health. The kidneys help maintain a balance of body fluids. The kidneys have the ability to filter out harmful toxic material while retaining the vital vitamins, proteins, sugars, fats and minerals. But if this system is overloaded with more toxins than it can eliminate, diseases will invade the body. It will cause protein in the blood to be lost in the urine. Potassium, calcium, magnesium and zinc can also be lost. This causes nutritional depletion and illness. Diseases associated with kidney failure are high blood pressure, stroke, heart attack or heart disease. It is important to protect the urinary system and nourish it with the proper food, vitamins, minerals, herbs and supplements that strengthen these vital organs.

URINARY FORMULA

The following nutrients strengthen the urinary system and prevent kidney and bladder problems.

Contains vitamins B_1—B_2—C—D—Folic Acid— Magnesium— Niacinamide—Pantothenic Acid—Potassium—

Uva Ursi—Hydrangea— Parsley—Dandelion—Siberian
Ginseng—Schizandra—Dong Quai— Cornsilk—Horsetail—
Hops—Lemon Bioflavonoids—

Special Urinary formulas

#1. This formula contains potassium and other essential
     minerals that are vital for urinary health.

     Kelp—Dulse—Watercress—Wild   Cabbage—
     Horseradish—Horsetail—

#2. This formula strengthens the urinary, reproductive,
     and digestive systems.

     Dong quai—Golden Seal—Juniper—Uva Ursi—
     Parsley—Ginger—Marshmallow—

#3. This formula provides nutrition for the urinary system.
     It will help protect the urinary organs from kidney
     stones, infections and water retention.

     Juniper Berries—Parsley—Uva Ursi—Dandlion—
     Chamomile—

#4. This formula strengthens the urinary system as well as
     the lymph system. This chinese formula contains the
     following.

     Stephania—Hoelen—Morus—Chaenomeles—
     Astragalus—Atryctylodes—Alisma—Magnolia—
     Polyporus—Areca—Aakebia—Cinnamon—Pinellis—
     Ginger—Citrus Peel—Licorice—

SINGLE HERBS FOR THE URINARY SYSTEM

Cornsilk—Garlic—Grapevine—Horsetail—
Hydrangea—Juniper Berries—Marshmallow—
Parsley—Peach Bark—Slippery Elm—Uva Ursi—

Bibliography

Airola, Paavo, Ph.D., N.D.
How To Get Well
Health Plus, Publisher, 1974

Bethel, May
The Healing Power of Herbs, 1969
The Healing Power of Natural Foods, 1978
Wilshire Book Co., No. Hollywood, Ca

Bianchini, Francesco, and **Corbetta, Francesco**
Health Plants of The World
Newsweek Books, New York

Bircher-Benner, M., M.D.
The Bircher-Benner Childrens Diet Book
Keats Publishing, Inc. 1977
New Canaan, Connecticut

Challen, Jack Joseph and **Renate Lewin**
What Herbs Are All About
Keats Publishing, Inc. 1980
New Canaan, Conn.

Christopher, Dr. John R.
The School of Natural Healing
BiWorld Publishers 1976

Clymer, R. Swinburne, M.D.
Nature's Healing Agents
The Humanitarian Society, First Printing 1905

Colby, Benjamin
Guide To Health, 1846 reprint
BiWorld Publisher, Orem, Utah

Coon, Nelson
Using Plants For Healing
Hearthside Press 1963
Rodale Press 1979

Culpeper, Nicholas
Culpepers' Herbal Remedies
Melvin Powers Wilshire Book Co., 1971
Culpepers Complete Herbal
W. Foulshan and Co., Ltd.

Dawson, Adele G.
Health, Happiness and The Pursuit of Herbs
The Stephen Greene Press, Vermont, 1980

Destreot, Raymond
Our Earth, Our Cure
Swan House Publishing Co, 1974

Farwell, Edith Foster
A Book of Herbs
The White Pine Press, 1979

Fluck, Prof. Hans
Medicinal Plants
Translated from German by Rowson, J. M.
W. Foulsham & Co., Ltd, England 1973

Gerard, John
The Herbal-The Complete 1633 Edition
Revised and Enlarged by Thomas Johnson
Dover Publications, Inc. New York 1975

Gibbons, Euell
Stalking The Wild Asparagus
David McKay Co., Inc. New York 1962

Graedon, Joe
The People's Pharmacy
Avon Publishers, New York 1980

Grieve, Mrs. M.
A Modern Herbal
Two Volumes: Dover Publications, Inc.

Griffin, LaDean
Is Any Sick Among You?
BiWorld Publisher, 1974

Harris, Ben Charles
The Complete Herbal
Larchmont Books, New York, 1972

Eat The Weeds
Keats Publishing, Inc., 1961

Hutchens, Alma R.
Indian Herbology of North America
Merco, 1973

Jensen, Dr. Bernard D. C.
Nature Has A Remedy, 1978

Kadans, Joseph, N. D., Phd.
Encyclopedia of Medicinal Herbs
Arco Publishing, Inc. New York 1970

Encyclopedia of Fruits, Vegetables, Nuts and Seeds for Healthful Living

Kirschmann, John D. Director
Nutrition Almanac, Revised Edition
McGraw-Hill Book Co. 1979

Kloss, Jethro
Back To Eden
Published and Distributed by the Jethro Kloss Family
Loma Linda, Ca.

Kordel, Lelord
Natural Fold Remedies
Manor Books, Inc. 1974

Krochmal, Arnold and **Connie**
A Guide to the Medicinal Plants of the United States
The New York Times Book Co. 1973

Kroeger, Hanna
Good Health Through Diets
Boulder, Colorado

Lewis, Walter H. and **Memory P. F. Elvin,**
Medical Botany-Plants Affecting Man's Health
John Wiley and Sons, New York

Malstrom, Dr. Stan N. D., M. T.
Own Your Own Body
Fresh Mountain Air Pub. Co. 1977
Herbal Remedies II revised
Woodland Books, 1975

McCleod, Dawn
Herb Handbook
Wilshire Book Co. 1968
No. Hollywood, Ca.

Merck Manual
Merck and Co., Inc. Ninth Edition

Meyer, Joseph E.
The Herbalist
Meyerbooks: copyright 1960

Montagna, F. Joseph
P.D.R.-Peoples Desk Reference
Vol I and II
Quest For Truth Publications, Inc.
Lake Oswego, Oregon 1979

Moore, Michael
Medicinal Plants of the Mountain West
The Museum of New Mexico Press, 1980

Pahlow, Mannfried
Living Medicine
Thorsons Publishers Limited-England 1980
First published in Germany 1976

Rau, Henrietta A. Diers
Healing With Herbs
Arco Publishing, Inc. New York 1976

Schauenberg, Paul and **Paris, Ferdinand**
Guide To Medicinal Plants
Keats Publishing, 1977

Shook, Dr. Edward E.
Elementary Treatise in Herbology-1974
Advanced Treatise in Herbology-1978
Trinity Center Press

Thomson, William A.R. M.D., Edited by,
Medicines From The Earth
McGraw-Hill Book Co. New York 1978

Tierra, Michael, C.A., N.D.
The Way of Herbs
Unity Press, Santa Cruz, 1980

United States Pharmacopeial Convention
The Physicians' and Pharmacists' Guide To Your Medicines
Ballantine Books-New York, 1981

Vogel, Alfred. Dr. h.c.
The Nature Doctor, 1952

Wade, Carlson
Bee Pollen and Your Health
Keats Publishing, Inc. Conn. 1978

Natural Hormones: The Secret of Youthful Health
Parker Publishing Co., Inc. New York, 1972

Wren, R. C.
Potter's New Cyclopedia of Medicinal Herbs and Preparations
Harper Colophon Books

Index

DIGESTION (ACIDS), herbs for 42
DIGESTION (PROMOTES), herbs for 104
DIGESTION AIDS, herbs for 149
DIGESTION PROMOTER, herbs for 46
DIGESTIVE PROBLEMS, herbs for 66, 71, 86
Digestive System, herbal formulas for 317-320
DIPHTHERIA, herbs for 11, 147
  treatment for 297
DISEASES, herbs for 56
DISINFECTANT HERBS 12
DIURETIC HERBS 19, 167
  herbal combinations for 219
DIVERTICULITIS, causes and treatment for 264
  herbs for 77, 113
DIZZINESS, herbs for 50, 74
Dong Quai, uses of 59
DROPSY, herbs for 83, 88, 106, 115
DRUG WITHDRAWAL, herbal combinations for 189
  herbs for 92
DRY SKIN, herbs for 290
DYSENTERY, causes and treatment for 264
  herbs for 22, 27, 30, 31, 99, 102, 144
DYSENTERY, ACUTE, herbs for 111

E

EAR AILMENTS, herbs for 130
EAR INFECTIONS, herbal combinations for 184
  herbs for 12, 18, 71, 73, 93, 130, 290
EARACHE, herbal combinations for 215
  herbs for 11, 50
  treatment for 297
EARACHE (OIL), herbs for 99
EARACHE (TINCTURE), herbs for 93
Echinacea, uses of 60
ECZEMA, herbal combinations for 171
  herbs for 11, 16, 30, 39, 89, 135, 136, 146
Elder Flower, uses of 61
Elecampane, uses of 62
Emergency Aids, herbs for 291-301
EMETIC HERBS 114
EMOTIONAL STRESS, herbs for 12
EMPHYSEMA, herbal combinations for 229
  herbs for 52, 57, 96, 111

ENDOCRINE GLANDS, herbs for 84
ENDURANCE, herbal combinations for 189, 200
  herbs for 57
ENDURANCE (INCREASES), herbs for 75
ENERGY, herbal combinations for 188, 200, 212
  herbs for 11, 28, 92, 161, 254, 261
ENERGY, INCREASES, herbs for 127
ENLARGED HEART, herbs for 80
ENVIRONMENTAL STRESS, herbs for 136
Enzymes, sources for 20, 25
Ephedra, uses of 62
EPIDEMICS, herbs for 23
EPILEPSY, causes and treatments for 261
  herbs for 32, 35, 93, 98, 128
ERUPTIONS, herbal combinations for 171
  herbs for 5, 82
ERYSIPELAS, herbal combinations for 171
Erythromycin, side effects of 216
Estrogen, side effects of 198, 233
Eucalyptus Oil, uses of 63, 304
Evening Primrose, uses of 64
EXCITABILITY, herbs for 123
EXHAUSTION, herbs for 23, 28
EXPECTORANT HERBS 61, 111, 143, 144
Extracts, as herbal preparations 3
EYE (STRENGTHENS), herbs for 65
EYE DISORDERS, herbs for 56
EYE INFECTIONS, herbs for 78, 94, 107
EYE INFLAMMATION, treatment for 297
EYE PROBLEMS, herbal combinations for 191
EYE TENSION, herbs for 107
EYE WASH, herbal combinations for 191
EYE, SORE, herbs for 134
Eyebright, uses of 65
EYELIDS, ULCERATED, herbs for 151
EYES (INFLAMMATION), herbs for 37

F

FALSE LABOR, causes and treatment for 284

1295